ALLERGY RELIEF

*Effective
Natural
Allergy
Treatments*

AVERY
a member of Penguin Putnam Inc.
New York

The information and procedures contained in this book are based on the research and the personal and professional experiences of the author. They are not intended as a substitute for consulting with your physician or other health-care provider. The publisher and the author are not responsible for any adverse effects or consequences resulting from the use of any of the suggestions, preparations, or procedures discussed in this book. All matters pertaining to your physical health should be supervised by a health-care professional. It is a sign of wisdom, not cowardice, to seek a second or third opinion.

Most Avery books are available at special quantity discounts for bulk purchase for sales promotions, premiums, fund-raising, and educational needs. Special books or book excerpts also can be created to fit specific needs. For details, write Putnam Special Markets, 375 Hudson Street, New York, NY 10014.

Avery
a member of
Penguin Putnam Inc.
375 Hudson Street
New York, NY 10014
www.penguinputnam.com

Library of Congress Cataloging-in-Publication Data

Goldfarb, Sylvia.
    Allergy relief : effective natural allergy treatments /
    Sylvia Goldfarb.
        p.   cm.
    Includes bibliographical references and index.
    ISBN 0-89529-997-6
    1. Allergy—Alternative treatment.   I. Title.
RC588.A47 G65   2000   00-020830
616.97'9206—dc21

Printed in the United States of America
10 9 8 7 6 5 4 3 2 1

This book is printed on acid-free paper. ∞

BOOK DESIGN BY RENATO STANISIC

COVER DESIGN BY KILEY THOMPSON

I dedicate this book to Mark G. Beals, my mentor, guide, and friend, for all his support, understanding, and patience in my sojourn through graduate school. This book would not exist if he had not recognized its potential when I submitted the introduction for my doctoral dissertation.

CONTENTS

ACKNOWLEDGMENTS

I am grateful to the following people for their help and support in the creation of this book.

Mark G. Beals, my mentor at Greenwich University, for realizing, upon receiving the opening chapters of what was intended to be my doctoral dissertation, the potential for a book and encouraging me to get it into the popular press.

Roberta Waddell, who edited my first two books at Instant Improvement and reviewed every word of this manuscript, for her valuable suggestions. And, for recommending me to Norman Goldfind at Avery.

Norman Goldfind, for calling me after reviewing the first few pages and telling me I had a publisher if I wanted to write the book. And, thank you again, Norman, for guiding me through the initial business aspects with the publisher.

Helene Ciaravino, for her positive strokes and for sending me helpful resource material.

Elaine Sparber, for her suggestions to improve the book as she meticulously reviewed the final manuscript line by line.

Dr. William L. Mundy, for giving me the idea for the initial project by presenting a seminar on treating allergies with visual imagery at the Ninth International Conference on the Psychology of Health, Immunity and Disease, given by the National Institute for the Clinical Application of Behavioral Medicine. Thank you again, Dr. Mundy, for always returning my calls and for sending me helpful material.

Dr. Edward M. Wagner, longtime friend and coauthor of my first two books, for always taking time from his busy schedule to answer questions and make sure that what I wrote was accurate.

Tom Wolfe and the rest of the staff at Smile Herb Shop in College Park, Maryland, for all their help and for sending me useful information.

All the physicians who helped me with this book, for graciously letting me interview them even though many of them wished to remain anonymous. It is my sincere hope that the day will come when they will feel free to lend their names to books on alternative healing.

Dorothy Pressman, my dear friend, for knowing when to encourage me to work and when to drag me away from my computer for some much needed rest and relaxation, and a few laughs. And thanks, Dottie, for your nurturing and letting me get so much work accomplished at your summer home.

Kali and Streaker, for sensing when the muse was sitting on my head and therefore snoozing quietly at my feet, then intuiting when I needed a break and taking me for a walk to clear my head.

And last, but certainly not least, Cookie, my bridegroom of thirty-nine years, for putting up with missed meals and unfolded laundry, and for checking everything I wrote to be sure it was clear and interesting, even to engineers and athletes.

FOREWORD

It has been my privilege to know Sylvia Goldfarb for a number of years. In this book, she focuses upon suggestions for taking charge of our health; on the fact that this may not be readily achieved, but that it can be achieved; that good health is a "state of being" that enriches all the dimensions of our lives.

This is a book worth our serious reading. Written in a warm, personable manner—almost as if we, the readers, were sitting across the table from the author, sharing a cup of coffee with her in her kitchen—it reflects some eighteen months of research of literature, interviews with members of the medical profession, and discussions with advocates of alternative remedies for health problems. From these endeavors has emerged scholarly, yet trustworthy and specific, advice. It is a book with vision. Sylvia sees that the "grassroots" movement of alternative medicine is beginning to gain momentum. She makes no effort to "fault" the medical profession, but, in the most scholarly manner possible, develops her position that alternative considerations must legitimately take their place beside establishment approaches. She insists, with documented justification, that there is a place for these alternatives.

For Sylvia, feeling energetic and healthy is the key to living well. In this excellent book, she has attempted to give us the gift of health. Join me in accepting that gift.

Mark G. Beals, PhD,
Dean, College of Social Science and Health,
Greenwich University, Norfolk Island, Australia

PREFACE

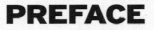

The inspiration for this book came from a seminar I attended on curing allergies with visual imagery that was given by William L. Mundy, MD. At the time, I was looking for a topic for my doctoral dissertation and submitted a proposal to my dissertation advisor for a paper comparing conventional and alternative allergy treatments. My advisor, Mark G. Beals, PhD, recognized the potential of the topic and suggested I write a book instead of a dissertation.

The purpose of the book that resulted—this book—is to enlighten readers about the various alternative methods for treating allergies so that they can make informed decisions as to which method or combination of methods would be best to use in their individual cases.

Those readers who seek more information on how to treat a particular condition—in this case, allergies—outside of mainstream medicine rarely have the time or inclination to first find individual books on each of the various alternative methods and to then look up each book's allergy section. It is yet more time-consuming and expensive to locate and consult a practitioner of each method. And, even if you do get that far, you do not end up with unbiased opinions, since most practitioners think that their method is the most effective, often to the exclusion of all the others. To save you all this work, I have done the research for you and present my findings in a clear, easy-to-understand fashion.

Although the treatment methods for allergies vary widely, most practitioners agree about the root cause of allergies—a malfunctioning or overreaction of the immune system. Before describing the various treatment methods, and to help you understand how they work, I therefore describe the immune system—what it is, how it works, and what can make it overreact. While both conventional and alternative practitioners agree about what causes allergies, they differ widely in their approaches to treating them.

This book was not written to denigrate the medical approaches to allergies, but rather to explain the various alternative approaches and to remind readers that they live in a free society and have the choice of how they wish to be treated.

I have tried to evenhandedly provide you with enough information about the current state of the art, including strengths and weaknesses, to help you select the best treatment, or combination of treatments, for your particular allergies.

Since all the treatments discussed in this book have both negative and positive aspects, I have included an appendix that allows you to quickly review the advantages and disadvantages of each treatment. There is also a section on resource organizations, listing phone numbers and websites, to help you locate more information on any of the therapies that interest you.

Taken together, the information in this book, in your hands, can spell the beginning of the end of your allergy problems.

ALLERGY RELIEF

INTRODUCTION

Do you or a family member suffer from allergies? Are you curious about the multitude of treatment methods available, but feel overwhelmed by all the information that is out there? Although most people are still not aware that methods outside of orthodox medical treatment exist, there is a growing recognition that alternative approaches may have positive outcomes for a high percentage of allergy patients. Alternative treatments, for the most part, are safe and non-toxic. More and more, these alternative methods are finding their way into mainstream medicine, and what was once dismissed as new-age nonsense is now being recognized as cutting-edge, safe therapy.

The various concepts of allergy treatment, both orthodox and alternative, are complex and broad. To get more information on these treatment methods, you would have to search for individual books on each approach, then look up each book's allergy section. Or, you would have to find and consult a practitioner of each of the methods, every one of whom most likely would think that his or her treatment was the most effective.

Here in this one book, on the other hand, you can conveniently find each available approach to allergy relief described in an informative, easy-to-understand, non-judgmental fashion. This book will equip you with the knowledge you need to become an informed consumer able to make an educated choice regarding how best to treat your allergies.

Before outlining the various treatment methods, however, I begin by describing, at length, in Chapter 1, just what an allergy is and how the immune system—there for protection—can make a mistake and initiate an allergic response. Chapter 1 also lists the most common causes of allergies and describes how allergies are often the unrecognized source of many illnesses.

The pros and cons of conventional therapies are described in Chapter 2, which also offers some very helpful advice about how to avoid exposing yourself to allergens. The medications currently in use, how they work, and their potential side effects are detailed.

In the first part of Chapter 3, you will learn about nutritional therapy, specifically which foods and beverages have therapeutic effects and which ones to avoid. The second part of the chapter deals with the benefits of nutritional supplements, suggests recommended dosages, and, where necessary, gives cautionary notes.

Herbal therapy, an ancient method of healing that is regaining popularity, is discussed in Chapter 4. Here you will find information about specific herbs that can provide relief from various types of allergies, along with instructions for preparing them.

Aromatherapy, the use of essential oils from plants, is sometimes considered a subspecialty of herbal therapy, but since it is gaining popularity as a useful complementary therapy, Chapter 5 is entirely devoted to it. In this chapter, you will learn how aromatherapy works and which oils and combinations are the most useful for treating allergies.

Homeopathy is a treatment method that defies all logic, yet it is the one that can best be tested by controlled studies. Chapter 6 fully describes the theory of homeopathy and gives its history. It answers the critics, describes the remedies, explains how to read the labels, and recommends which of the remedies to take to relieve your allergies.

Three types of energy balancing—acupuncture, acupressure, and reflexology—are detailed in Chapter 7. You are probably aware of them for pain control, but did you know they also can be used to treat allergies and asthma?

Nambudripad's Allergy Elimination Techniques (NAET) is a revolutionary approach for allergy treatment that, in many cases, achieves permanent allergy relief by reprogramming the immune system. Although it is somewhat time-consuming and expensive, patients are thrilled with its results. Chapter 8 describes this method and includes several case histories.

Chapter 9 is about another unusual method for allergy treatment—visual imagery, the method that was the original impetus for this book. You may have heard about the visualization process being used to control pain and to help stimulate the immune systems of cancer patients, but did you know that it can also be used to retrain the immune system not to react to allergy-causing substances?

Knowledge is power, and it is my hope that this book will enlighten you about the various forms of allergy treatments, while emphasizing the safest, drug-free options, so that you can make an educated choice as to which treatments are best for you.

Allergy Relief: Effective Natural Allergy Treatments brings you from symptoms to solutions to help you feel better every single day!

1

Defining and Diagnosing Allergies

An allergy is an abnormal and inappropriate response by the immune system to a substance that is not normally harmful to people. The immune system mistakenly identifies a non-toxic substance as an invader, and the allergic response itself becomes a disease. Allergic responses often include symptoms such as nasal congestion, watery eyes, wheezing, coughing, itching, hives, rash, headache, and fatigue.

Allergies can produce symptoms in every organ of the body, and they often masquerade as other diseases. They can affect the nose, throat, eyes, ears, lungs, digestive tract, bladder, vagina, skin, muscles, joints, and entire nervous system, including the brain. The substances that cause allergies are called *antigens,* and they are different for every person. Special types of antigens called *allergens* stimulate a particular antibody, immunoglobulin E, or IgE, into response. An IgE response, then, is due to the overproduction of a specific antibody. Cellular allergy is the other type of response and is caused when the lymphocytes, or lymph cells, which function in the body's immune response, overreact to rid the body of a foreign material. This is the response by which the body rejects transplanted organs.

Of the millions of people who suffer from allergies, some experience only mild symptoms, while others have serious symptoms that can weaken their internal organs and compromise their immune systems. For example, *anaphylactic shock* is a severe, sudden allergic reaction characterized by choking, a drop in the blood pressure, heart failure, and even, in catastrophic cases, death.

Undiagnosed allergies can lead to illnesses and chronic diseases that can affect every part of the body. Therefore, it is important that you learn as much as you can about allergies and how to alleviate them. This chapter presents basic information on the various types of allergies and how they are diagnosed. Also discussed is the bodily system behind allergies—the immune system.

THE IMMUNE SYSTEM AND ALLERGIES

The function of the immune system is to protect the body from harmful invaders, but in the case of allergies, it takes unnecessary measures and carries out defense mechanisms against substances that are harmless. The body goes into a heightened state of alert— the blood vessels dilate; the nerves stand on end, causing itching;

and adrenaline and histamine flood the system. In most allergic reactions, the white blood cells overreact, and the allergic response itself becomes a disease.

For example, you may have had an infection, cold, or sore throat at the same time that you had some tiny particles (allergens) present in your bloodstream. Prior to the infection, these tiny particles had always been handled by your lymph glands and macrophage cells (special cells that protect the body against infection), which simply washed the particles out of your body. But when your immune cells were busy attacking the bacteria or viruses of your infection, they identified the innocuous particles as another type of foreign body and placed markers on them, too. Then, in about five days, your body produced special cells (antigens) to attack all the marked particles. Now, whenever your body senses the presence of the innocuous particles, the antigens come out in force to attack them. As stated by William L. Mundy, MD, clinical professor of medicine at the University of Missouri School of Medicine, Kansas City, "The immune system treats tourists as if they were terrorists." Histamine is released at the site where the immune cells attack the allergen, and it is this histamine that causes the symptoms associated with allergies—inflammation, congestion, and mucus.

Clemens Von Perquet, an Austrian pediatrician, created the word "allergy" in 1906 by combining two Greek words—*allos,* which means "altered," and *ergion,* which refers to "action" or "reactivity." In 1921, two German scientists discovered what causes these "altered reactions." Carl Prausnitz and Heinz Kustner conducted an experiment when Dr. Kustner developed hives shortly after eating fish. In the experiment, blood serum from Dr. Kustner was injected into Dr. Prausnitz's arm. The next day, fish extract was injected in the same place on Dr. Prausnitz's arm. The result was an inflamed, itchy bump. Dr. Prausnitz and Dr. Kustner named the unknown component in the blood that caused the allergic reaction a *reagin.* The Prausnitz-Kustner test, or *positive-transfer test,* was used to diagnose allergies for a number of years.

Decades later, in the United States during the 1960s, a husband-and-wife scientific team, Kimishige and Teruko Ishizaka, discovered that reagins are a form of IgE, the antibody most frequently involved in immediate allergic reactions. Allergy-prone people produce an overabundance of antibodies, which in turn trigger the mast cells (histamine-containing cells found in the mucous membranes, skin, and bronchial tubes) to release the inflammation-causing histamines and leukotrienes. The goal of antibodies is to fight infection. The major antibodies are immunoglobulin A (IgA), immunoglobulin E (IgE), immunoglobulin G (IgG), and immunoglobulin M (IgM). Allergic individuals have much higher concentrations of IgE, and all individuals produce IgE antibodies specific to their allergens.

IgE is formed as part of an allergic response. The allergic response can take place anywhere in the body and can cause severe problems. When IgE is produced in the lung tissue, the result is shortness of breath or asthma. When it is produced in the skin, the outcome is hives. In the wall of the intestinal tract, IgE causes gas, pain, and/or bloating. In the head, it can induce swelling of the lining of the brain, which can lead to a drastic condition such as schizophrenia or violent aggression.

COMMON ALLERGENS

Although allergies can stem from anything, the substances that most commonly set off false alarms in the immune system are seasonal factors such as pollen, mold, and grass; dust; certain metals; cosmetics; lanolin; insect bites; foods; common drugs; cleaning products; air pollutants such as asbestos, smoke, and fumes; and dander from animals. Less common allergens are tobacco smoke, gas for cooking and heating, and the metals used by dentists to fill teeth.

As previously stated, substances that cause allergies are called allergens. For the purpose of convenience, these substances have been divided into five categories. These categories are inhalants, ingestants, contactants, injectants, and molds and fungi.

Inhalants

Inhalants are allergens that are drawn into the body through the nose or throat. Examples are pollen, grass, and flower spores; and smoke, perfume, and chemical fumes. The allergic symptoms provoked by inhalants include runny nose, sneezing, coughing, wheezing, sinus congestion, and watery, itchy eyes.

Two types of inhalant allergies are hay fever and allergic rhinitis (inflammation of the mucous membrane lining the nose). They are often confused with each other because their symptoms are very similar. "Hay fever" is an old term for a seasonal reaction to pollen and molds. It has nothing to do with hay and does not cause a fever. A nineteenth-century physician created the term when he sneezed after entering his hay-filled barn and misdiagnosed the cause of his allergy. What we call hay fever usually occurs during the spring, summer, and fall, while allergic rhinitis is more year-round, usually caused by mold, dust, feathers, fur, chalk, or animal dander. (For a discussion of allergy to animal dander, see "Why Cats Are More Often the Culprit" on the next page.) Some people suffer from both hay fever and allergic rhinitis.

Why Cats Are More Often the Culprits

The reason more people are allergic to cats than to dogs is that allergy to animal fur is really allergy to dander. Dander is loose, scaly dry skin, which animals spread over their bodies via their saliva. Animals deposit their saliva on their coats while cleaning themselves. And we all know that cats preen more than dogs. Therefore, cats have more dander spread over their bodies, which means they have more dander ready to be inhaled by allergic individuals. Fortunately for allergic animal lovers, there are sprays and solutions that can be applied to animals' fur to reduce the dander and make it possible to enjoy those adorable creatures.

Ingestants

Ingestants are allergens that are taken into the body through the mouth as food. They can have a wide range of effects on the body. Some ingestants can negatively affect the gastrointestinal system, others can wreak havoc on the skin, and still others can trigger problems with the body's most basic functions, such as breathing and heart rhythm. Besides resulting from the consumption of specific foods, food allergies also can be caused by food-related factors such as poor nutrition. For more information on defining and diagnosing food allergies, see "More About Food Allergies" on page 16.

Contactants

Contactants are allergens that cause a reaction when they come into direct contact with the skin. Some common contactants are poison ivy, poison oak, poison sumac, cosmetics, detergents, chemicals, and latex. The most common symptoms of skin allergies are redness, hives, itching, dermatitis, and rash. The severity of the reaction can range from merely annoying to severe enough to impair sleep. For the most part, skin allergies are not life-threatening, but hives in the area of the throat or mouth could interfere with breathing and/or swallowing.

Injectants

Injectants are exactly what they sound like—allergens that are injected into the body. They include the poisons from insect bites, as well as substances that medicine relies on to encourage better health, such as vaccines, serums, drugs, and antitoxins. The reaction can be localized, in the form of a small or large itchy spot or bump accompanied by some redness of the skin, or it can be systemic, in the form of hives or generalized itching. In rare cases, the reaction can be life-threatening, such as when the throat tissues swell severely enough to interfere with breathing.

Molds

Molds are microscopic fungi (plants lacking chlorophyll) that live on plant or animal matter, which they decompose for their sustenance. In order to reproduce, they release spores into the air that fall on the organic matter and grow into new mold clusters. Airborne mold spores are far more prevalent than pollen grains and can enter the body in a number of ways. They can be injected, inhaled, ingested, or touched. Molds can cause a variety of nasal symptoms and are a prime source of irritation for asthmatics.

FACTORS THAT CAUSE ALLERGIES

Some people are born allergic to certain substances. Others develop allergies over a period of time or as a result of a significant experience with a substance. The factors that cause allergies can be narrowed down to several categories—heredity, environment, medications and immunizations, stress, and nutrition.

Heredity

Heredity is a major factor in developing allergic reactions. The more relatives people have with allergies, the earlier in life they will experience their own allergic manifestations. Allergies tend to run in families because the tendency to produce higher concentrations of IgE is inherited. When IgE antibodies form in the blood and circulate throughout the body, an individual becomes sensitized to the allergen. The sensitization process can happen quickly, after only a single exposure, or gradually, over a period of many years. Heredity causes some people to have a highly sensitive system from the very beginning. A few people are born with responses to allergens that are akin to jumping out of the skin when touched only lightly on the shoulder.

Environment

In today's polluted world, the toxic load on our systems is increasing to the point that impaired immune response from toxic overload is now recognized as one of the primary causes of allergies. Indoor pollution is a serious problem that can be caused by fumes from carpeting, paint, telephone and television cables, and formaldehyde. Other indoor household irritants are cleaning products, aerosol sprays, disinfectants, and air fresheners. Many office buildings are constructed in an energy-saving fashion and are so tightly sealed that they have a serious lack of ventilation. The indoor pollutants in these buildings are so widespread that symptoms relating to them are known as sick-building syndrome. You can't even escape from environmental pollutants in your car, since it also is filled with all sorts of irritants, such as carpeting, plastic, and leather.

But the environment does not have to be laden with chemicals and soot to irritate the body. The most natural of landscapes can also provoke allergies, due to such elements as pollen and poisonous plants. And if you change locations, new environmental factors can trigger allergic responses. For example, natives of the southwestern region of the United States have to contend with new airborne, waterborne, and foodborne substances if they move to the northeast and their immune systems do not adjust well.

Immunizations and Medications

Charles Gableman, MD, a practitioner of environmental medicine in California, believes that immunizations and overprescribed medications are two primary causes of allergies. He counsels that vaccine shots actually disturb the immune systems of infants. Some babies react more severely than others, depending on factors such as heredity and nutrition. This issue has many parents seeking out as much information as possible before deciding whether or not to have their newborns immunized with routine boosters.

Dr. Gableman also reports that the overprescribing of antibiotics and steroids damages the intestinal flora. Antibiotics can confuse the immune system until it can no longer tell friend from foe. When this happens, the immune system reacts negatively to harmless, friendly substances. Pain, gas, bloating, and even bleeding can result.

Many people find that they are allergic to certain drugs. Drug reactions can range from minor (a brief skin rash) to fatal. There is no consistency in the reactions to certain medications. Penicillin, for example, has saved countless lives, yet many people have had devastating reactions to it and do not leave the house in the morning without an identification bracelet that states, "Allergic to penicillin." Medications are potent substances that can manipulate the body's natural immune reactions. It is not surprising that they sometimes result in allergies.

Nutrition

Many health problems, such as headaches, abdominal distress, and skin eruptions, are directly related to undiagnosed food allergies, and it is possible that what you eat could be a major factor in your allergies. For a detailed discussion of food allergies, see "More About Food Allergies" on page 16. For a complete discussion of nutritional therapy, see Chapter 3.

Stress

Stressful lifestyles also result in the body having a reduced immune response and an inability to cope with allergens. Stress of all kinds—negative and positive, emotional and physical—can lead to the development of allergies. Many people find that after a traumatic incident their immune system no longer functions optimally and allergies develop. Examples of such traumatic incidents are a major illness, the death of a loved one, the loss of a job, a car accident, and a physical affront such as a mugging. Many people feel that if they had not experienced the major trauma, their allergies might not have developed.

Dr. William Mundy explains that white blood cells, which protect the body from harmful organisms such as bacteria and viruses, increase in total number when fighting infection and also when the organism is operating under stressful, acute physical conditions. In fact, they can change their number and activities even when you are simply contemplating a stressful situation. This shows that stress greatly affects the immune system and, therefore, its response to foreign entities that can become allergens. The average life span of a white blood cell is five to eight weeks, and the body constantly produces new ones. Each new cell generation is somehow passed the information it needs to maintain the immune response, and Dr. Mundy believes that the mind is the reason.

THE SKIN AND ALLERGIES

Allergies are often the unrecognized causes of many modern illnesses. Most allergens produce congestion symptoms, as the body attempts to seal them off from its regular processes or tries to work around them. When an allergen invades the body, extra mucus forms a shield around it, leading to sinus congestion, stuffy nose, headache, and watery eyes. And when the body attempts to eliminate the excess congestion through the skin, a rash, fever blister, abscess, and/or sore throat can develop. Since the skin is the body's largest organ of elimination and is an indicator of what's going on *inside* the body, it's a good idea to take skin eruptions seriously. The three most common skin allergies are contact dermatitis, eczema, and hives.

Contact dermatitis is purely an external condition, caused by physical contact with an allergen. It is localized and confined to the area that was directly exposed to the offending substance. This skin allergy can be resolved quite easily simply by avoiding the allergen.

Eczema is an inflammation of the skin characterized by symptoms such as scaling, crusting, and blistering. It is a chronic skin disease that occurs most often in people who suffer from food allergies and nutritional deficiencies. Although it is unsightly, it is not contagious.

Hives can be caused by cold weather, sun exposure, medications, hidden food allergies, or chronic candidiasis (a yeast infection caused by an impaired immune system, antibiotics, anti-inflammatory drugs, or immunosuppressive drugs). Hives are the most serious of the three types of common skin allergies. For example, in the mouth and throat, hives can block the breathing passages and become life-threatening.

If you notice episodes of rashes, irritation, or hives, see a dermatologist. The skin tells an important story, giving you external signs of what you otherwise can't see. As already mentioned, you may simply have touched something that you shouldn't, but you also may have severe nutritional issues or immune resistances that need to be addressed.

MORE ABOUT FOOD ALLERGIES

When Hippocrates, the Father of Medicine, wrote that he noticed cheese caused an adverse reaction in some people, he became the first person ever to record an allergic reaction to food. James Braly, MD, medical director of Immune Labs, Fort Lauderdale, Florida, believes that food allergies, along with deficiencies in bodily nutrition and faulty assimilation of food, are the most frequently undiagnosed conditions in the United States. The foods that most commonly cause reactions are eggs, dairy products, wheat, peanuts, soybeans, chicken, fish, mollusks and shellfish, nuts, tomatoes, and corn.

Effects on the Body

The primary target for food allergies is the gastrointestinal system. After a food that offends the system is ingested, the result may be abdominal distention, cramps, gas, diarrhea, nausea, and/or vomiting. Reactions can occur quickly, often when the food is still in the mouth, even before it has traveled down to the stomach and intestines.

The skin is also a target. Adverse reactions can range from simple itching to severe, giant hives (angioedema). Itching, as well as swelling of the lips, throat, and oral mucous membranes may be experienced as soon as the food is ingested. In addition, food allergies can lead to flare-ups of asthma, eczema, or rhinitis, especially in children. Anyone with a personal or family history of asthma, hay fever, or eczema is at a somewhat greater risk for food allergies.

The most common symptoms of food allergies are runny nose, abdominal discomfort, skin eruptions, and depression. If not taken seriously, they can result in reactions such as anaphylactic shock.

Hidden Triggers

If you have identified specific whole foods that irritate you, your best bet is simply to eliminate those foods from your diet. But often, food allergies are triggered by common ingredients within foods. For instance, caramel coloring, xanthan gum, lecithin, modified food starch, citric acid, and malto-dextrin are all corn-derived additives, and corn is a common allergy producer. Even the glue on postage stamps is coated with a corn derivative.

Besides being induced by foods, food allergies can be caused by nutritional deficiencies. A diet that is too repetitive can cause food allergies. Also, pesticides and preservatives in the food chain can irritate and sicken people. Food additives such as artificial sweeteners, flavor enhancers, and colorants can cause reactions that range from mild to life-threatening. Finally, intestinal-yeast overgrowth can cause unhealthy gut conditions that result in food allergies. A diet of healthy, whole foods that were organically grown is ideal. However, the reality is that many of us don't have the time for, money for, or access to such a health-conscious diet. But we can try (as every effort counts), and most of us can do better than we are doing. Just becoming more aware of what we ingest is the first step.

Food Allergy Versus Food Intolerance

There is a difference between food allergy and food intolerance. A food intolerance does not involve the immune system, while a food allergy does. Food intolerance, or sensitivity, involves only the body's metabolism. In food intolerance, the body lacks an enzyme needed to digest a particular food, but the immune system is not compromised.

It is possible to have a combination of an immune-system dysfunction and a metabolic disorder. This dual food-related problem can lead to *leaky gut syndrome,* in which undigested food particles (fats, proteins, starches, and even bacteria) normally eliminated in the urine and feces are instead absorbed into the system. This unhealthy absorption is due to chronic irritation of the intestinal lining. Toxicity and a weakened immune system result, increasing vulnerability to allergies. It's a truly vicious cycle.

Diagnoses of Food Allergies

There are two ways to diagnose a food allergy—the elimination diet and the pulse test. An *elimination diet* should be closely supervised by an alternative-healthcare practitioner. If you suffer any type of illness while you're on this diet, you must stop, treat the ailment, and then start over when you are feeling better.

The elimination diet is a fairly simple diet. First, for seven to ten days, you eat foods that are unlikely to cause an allergic reaction—for example, rice, fruit, meat, and certain vegetables. Then, you slowly add new foods, one at a time, one day at a time. If you react to any food, make a note of your symptoms and wait at least twenty-four to forty-eight hours before introducing another food. By keeping track of which foods cause a reaction, you will know which foods to avoid.

The *pulse test* is a quicker diagnostic tool. You simply avoid a particular food for four days. Then, you take your pulse, eat the food by itself, wait twenty minutes, and take your pulse again. If your heart rate has gone up or down by ten beats per minute, you may be allergic to the food.

Once you have identified your allergies, your main goal will be to devise a nutritional plan that avoids the irritating foods while providing optimal nutrition. For information on preventing food-allergy attacks through nutrition, see Chapter 2.

DIAGNOSIS OF ALLERGIES

A doctor might suspect that you have an allergy if you report that your cold has lasted for an extended length of time. You assume it is a cold because your nose is clogged and runny, and you have to blow it so often that your social life is impaired. In addition, your eyes tear and itch, your sleep is disturbed, and you can't concentrate. Doesn't that sound like a cold? It could be an allergy instead.

When you go to the doctor, you first will be questioned to determine if your symptoms include fever, body aches, discolored nasal discharge, and/or coughing, all symptoms of a cold rather than an allergy. The physician will then complete a history and will most likely ask you the following questions:

- When did your symptoms first appear?
- Where were you when they first appeared and what were you doing?
- What type of work do you do?
- What are your hobbies?
- Do you have any pets?

By carefully questioning you, the doctor can reduce the list of suspected allergens and thereby limit the number of allergy tests to a manageable level. Among the diagnostic tests generally used today are skin tests and blood tests.

Skin Testing

Your doctor will probably suggest skin testing first, as it is a simple, reliable, and relatively inexpensive method that produces immediate results. The types of skin tests are the scratch test, the prick test, the intradermal test, and the patch test.

The *scratch test* consists of applying small dilutions of suspected allergens, such as dust mites, pollens, and molds, to tiny scratches made on the skin, usually on the forearm. If itching, reddening, or swelling appear within fifteen to thirty minutes, an allergy to the test substance is suspected.

The *prick test* is similar to the scratch test, but instead of applying the suspected allergen to a scratch, a drop of an extract of the allergen is placed on the skin and a needle is passed through the extract to make a tiny puncture in the skin. The extract then seeps into the skin, and the doctor watches for a reaction.

Some practitioners believe the *intradermal test* is more accurate than the scratch or prick test. For the intradermal test, a small amount of the allergen extract is injected into the top layer of the skin to see if symptoms appear.

Finally, the *patch test* is usually used to look for substances causing contact dermatitis. The suspected allergen is placed on the skin and covered with a bandage for forty-eight hours. An allergy is indicated if the skin becomes reddened or peels.

Be sure to tell your doctor if you are taking an antihistamine because it can interfere with skin testing. You will probably have to stop taking the antihistamine for a specific period of time before undergoing the testing. For some people, skin testing should not be performed at all. The two main reasons are the presence of a widespread skin condition or eczema, or the possibility of being so sensitive to the allergen that the testing could be dangerous.

Blood Testing

A more expensive but safer test is the *radioallergosorbent test (RAST)*, a blood test. After a sample of blood is drawn, drops of it are mixed with various allergens and examined under a microscope for the degree of allergic reaction. This test is not affected by medications. In addition, it is safer because it induces the allergic reaction outside of the body, using simply blood cells.

Allergies can be caused by a number of factors, and they can be stubborn problems. In addition, just as the causes of allergies are many and varied, so are the approaches to treating them. The following chapters will address these approaches. Some of the approaches may be familiar to you, while others are on the cutting edge and may be new to you.

2

Conventional Therapies

If your doctor suspects your problems are caused by allergies, he or she will probably refer you to a specialist for diagnosis and treatment. Physicians who specialize in treating allergies are known as allergists or clinical immunologists. If you test positive for allergies, your doctor will recommend one or a combination of the following three strategies—avoidance, medications, and immunotherapy (shots).

AVOIDANCE

Once the cause of your allergy has been identified, your first step should be to decrease or eliminate your exposure to the allergen. This means that you will have to better control your environment. Allergen avoidance is the ideal solution.

Avoiding Inhalants

Many allergy sufferers consider moving to a different location, yet allergists seldom recommend this as a cure for allergies. You may escape from one substance to which you are allergic—ragweed, for example—and then develop a sensitivity to another substance in the new location—grasses, for example.

Pollen, dander, mold, and dust mites are difficult to avoid entirely, but the following suggestions will help reduce your exposure to them:

- Keep your windows closed, and use an air conditioner with a high-energy particulate air (HEPA) filter to help clean the pollen and mold from indoor air.
- Use the air conditioner in your automobile.
- Don't hang clothing out to dry because pollen clings to fabric.
- Limit the time you spend outdoors between 5 and 10 A.M., when the air is most saturated with pollen.
- If you mow your own lawn or work in your garden, take your allergy medication before you start and wear a dust mask while you work.
- Use a damp cloth when dusting, and vacuum frequently. Ideally, you should have someone else do the cleaning, but if this is impossible, wear a dust mask.

- Get rid of your carpeting, as it is a breeding ground for dust mites. If you must have some carpeting, use rugs that can be washed weekly.
- Use wooden, leather, or vinyl-covered furniture rather than upholstered chairs and sofas.
- Use closed cabinets rather than open shelves.
- Cover your windows with washable curtains or window shades rather than heavy drapes or venetian blinds.
- Change or clean the filters in your air conditioner and furnace often.
- When you don't run your air conditioner, use a HEPA air cleaner. This is a device that can remove particles as small as .01 micron, which are a thousand times smaller than the smallest dust particles visible to the naked eye.
- Cover your mattress and pillow with allergen-proof plastic.
- Wash your bedding weekly.
- Use a vacuum cleaner with an efficient filtering unit that will not spread allergens through the air.
- Keep your pets out of your bedroom.
- Keep a nightlight on in dark closets to reduce the growth of mold and mildew.
- If your child plays with stuffed animals, bag and store the toys in the freezer between play sessions. This will kill the dust mites.
- Use an exhaust fan in your bathroom while you shower to reduce the mold buildup.

These suggestions are easy to follow and are also relatively inexpensive.

Avoiding Contactants

All sorts of contactants can cause skin reactions, but by exercising a minimal amount of caution, you can prevent many problems.

If you suspect your cosmetics or bath products are causing your skin problems, use hypo-allergenic products. It is always a good idea to perform a skin test with new brands before using them. Apply a small amount to the inner surface of your arm, cover the area, and check it in twenty-four hours. If any redness or itching is present, don't use the product. It is especially important to perform a skin test if you dye your hair. Even a different color within the same brand can cause a reaction.

Sometimes, the gloves you use to protect your hands from chemicals can cause a problem. For example, you may develop an allergy to the latex in the gloves. If this occurs, try using cotton-lined gloves.

Synthetic fabrics can cause problems. In addition, some natural fabrics, such as wool, may not affect you outdoors in cool weather, but may cause you to react when you are indoors, where it is warm.

Learn to recognize and avoid poisonous plants. These can be found both outdoors and indoors.

If you have a stubborn skin problem that doesn't seem to have an apparent cause, try changing your laundry detergent or fabric softener. Many people are sensitive to some brands of these products, but do well with others.

People who tend to have allergic skin reactions need to be aware of everything, especially new items that come into contact with their body. Learn to take note of your surroundings and to handle new items with care.

Avoiding Ingestants

In addition to avoiding the whole foods that cause you to have an allergic reaction, you have to beware of foods that have been genetically engineered. For instance, you may be allergic to Brazil nuts, but feel safe consuming soybean products. What you may not be aware of is that, in an attempt to improve the protein quality of soybeans, scientists have transplanted genetic material from Brazil nuts into them. Therefore, you also need to be careful eating soybean products, since genetically altered soybeans could cause you to suffer allergic reactions. Similarly, if you have an allergy to corn, you must avoid consuming baked goods containing high-fructose corn syrup.

A recent study suggested that about 5 percent of the American population may suffer from adverse reactions to food. If you are allergic to a particular food, you may be allergic to related foods—that is, foods in the same botanical family. For example, if you are allergic to avocados, you may also react to bay leaves, since they are a member of the same plant family as avocados. If you are allergic to peanuts, you may react when you eat peas, beans, or licorice, which are also in the legume family.

Irwin G., an electrical contractor, had always liked fruit, but he started to flush and develop a tingling sensation in his mouth and throat after eating apples, peaches, plums, and cherries. Fearful of a more severe reaction, he stopped eating all fruit. Then, one day, he mentioned to his wife, a horticulture student, that almonds also caused a reaction. Mrs. G. knew that almonds, apples, peaches, plums, and cherries all belong to the rose family, along with pears and nectarines. Fortunately, Mr. G. just needed to eliminate this one family of fruits from his diet and could still enjoy melons, citrus fruits, and berries.

Sometimes, a food allergy is triggered by a seasonal allergy. For example, your pollen allergy may trigger an allergy to eggs. Therefore, you may not be able to eat eggs in the summer even though you can eat them safely at all other times of the year.

If you have a food allergy, you must check ingredients very carefully to be sure that an offending food or food additive is not present. And, if you have food allergies, *never* lick the glue on envelopes or stamps. Some glues are made from fish products or plant products and can cause you to have an allergic reaction. Also, never take even a taste of any food that has given you a severe, immediate reaction, as this could provoke a life-threatening response.

If you have more mast cells than normal, you are more prone to allergies than the average person, so you should avoid the following food additives, which increase the production of a compound that increases the number of mast cells in the body:

- Colorings (azo dyes) and yellow dye number 5 (tartrazine).
- Flavorings (salicylates, aspartame).
- Preservatives (benzoates, nitrites, sorbic acid).
- Synthetic antioxidants (hydroxytoluene, sulfite, gallate).
- Emulsifiers/stabilizers (polysorbates, vegetable gums).

Once a diagnosis of a food allergy is made, the only proven therapy is strict elimination of the offending substance. Therefore, you must carefully scrutinize food labels for potential sources of food allergens.

Avoiding Injectants

The toxins delivered by biting insects are injectants, so if you are allergic to injectants, you need to avoid being bitten by bugs. To this end, you should never wear perfume or fragrant lotions, or brightly colored clothing. Avoid places that stinging insects habituate, such as marshes, flowerbeds, and areas near garbage. Always wear shoes when you walk in grass.

Avoid anything that makes you *smell* like a flower, such as perfume, scented soap, after-shave lotion, or suntan lotion. Avoid anything that makes you *look* like a flower, such as flowered or brightly colored clothing. At the same time, don't wear dark colors such as brown, black, or navy because these colors also might provoke an attack. Bees are least attracted to light khaki and white.

MEDICATIONS

Although the ideal way to prevent allergies is to avoid offending substances, it is almost impossible to fully implement this. Instead, your doctor will most likely advise you to use over-the-counter remedies or prescription medications to help relieve your symptoms.

Antihistamines

Antihistamines, first developed by French scientists in the late 1930s, are the least expensive and most commonly used treatment for allergies. Antihistamines do not block the release of histamine, as is commonly thought. Instead, they block the action of the histamine on the affected tissues. They help dry excess secretions and reduce itching and sneezing, but they don't do much for nasal congestion. Although they do reduce symptoms, they are not a cure for allergies.

Several classes of antihistamines are available, and some can be purchased without a doctor's prescription. The most common antihistamines in this category are:

- Brompheniramine (Dimetapp, Dimetane, Drixoral).
- Chlorpheniramine (Allerest, Chlor-Trimeton, Coricidin, Triaminic).
- Diphenhydramine (Benadryl).
- Phenyltoloxamine (Sinutab).

Except for causing drowsiness and some dryness, antihistamines are relatively safe. They can have some other side effects, however, including urinary retention in men with enlarged prostates and the possible aggravation of glaucoma. Moreover, antihistamines occasionally do more harm than good because they thicken the mucus, which prevents it from draining. Thickened mucus can stagnate, encouraging bacterial growth. If you have nasal dryness or thickened mucus, you should avoid taking antihistamines.

Drowsiness is the principal side effect of antihistamines. As little as 50 milligrams of Benadryl can impair your driving by as much as a 0.1-blood-alcohol content. You also should be aware that alcohol and tranquilizers increase the sedative effect of antihistamines. In fact, the older (first-generation) antihistamines just listed have such strong sedative effects that the major over-the-counter sleeping aids are derived from them.

At one time, people with allergic rhinitis were disqualified from working as pilots on the grounds that either their medication or their allergy symptoms could interfere with their performance. Prior to the advent of second-generation (non-sedating) antihistamines, many patients chose to endure their symptoms rather than put up with the adverse effects of these drugs. Second-generation, non-sedating antihistamines, available by prescription only, include:

- Terfenadine (Seldane).
- Fexofenadine hydrochloride (Allegra).
- Astemizole (Hismanal).
- Loratadine (Claritin).
- Ceterizine (Zyrtec).

Seldane was introduced in 1985 and promoted as the first allergy treatment that does not cause drowsiness. By 1995, wholesale sales totaled $400 million. In 1996, there were 4.3 million prescriptions written for Seldane and 2.3 million for Seldane-D. (*Note:* When the name of an antihistamine is followed by the letter "D," it means that a decongestant has been added.)

When these non-sedating antihistamines were first introduced, they were regarded as panaceas, but they are not without side effects. A minor effect of second-generation antihistamines is weight gain, but there are also other, more serious risks, such as cardiovascular problems. In addition, non-sedating antihistamines can interact dangerously with other drugs.

As of May 1992, fifteen deaths have been linked to Seldane and Hismanal. In 1993, the Food and Drug Administration (FDA) began receiving reports of cardiac arrhythmia in patients with liver disease and in those taking Seldane along with certain other drugs, such as the antibiotic erythromycin or the anti-fungal agent ketoconazole. On December 29, 1997, the manufacturer of Seldane said it would voluntarily remove the product from the marketplace by February 1, 1998, in response to the FDA's approval of the company's safer alternative drug, Allegra. The drug Hismanal, manufactured by a different company, has been shown to have the same heart risks as Seldane, and it, too, should be removed from circulation.

Drug interactions can be dangerous. During a twenty-two-month period, 122 reactions occurred in patients taking Seldane or Hismanal along with an antibiotic or anti-fungal medication. In almost half these instances, the patients had obtained their prescriptions from different physicians. In one case in particular, a fifty-two-year-old hospital technician was given a prescription for erythromycin by one physician and, three days later, was given a prescription for Seldane by another physician. After taking both drugs for four days, she experienced sudden dizziness and blurred vision. She was fortunate in that the episode occurred at the hospital where she worked because she was immediately monitored and treated with lidocaine, intravenous magnesium, and the temporary implantation of a transvenous pacemaker. She eventually recovered.

Amy Kaufman was not so fortunate. The wife of a neurosurgeon, she was having trouble with hives and, as instructed by her dermatologist, had been taking one tablet of Hismanal every morning. One night after dinner, when her hives were still bothering her, she asked her husband if he thought it would be all right for her to take one extra tablet of Hismanal. He replied, "One tablet can't kill you." The next morning, however, she was dead in the bed next to him. The autopsy report said her death was caused by cardiac arrest and implicated the Hismanal. This was so traumatic for Dr. Kaufman that he ended up abandoning his practice of medicine.

Decongestants

Oral decongestants are available over the counter and by prescription. Decongestants, also known as vasoconstrictors, work by constricting the tiny blood vessels in the affected areas. They do not cause grogginess, but may cause an increase in blood pressure, dizziness, headaches, and nervousness. Sudafed is one of the best-known oral decongestants.

During severe allergy attacks, topical decongestants, such as Neosinephrine and Afrin nose drops, go to work quickly. They temporarily open nasal passages for several hours. However, they should not be used for more than five consecutive days because a tolerance may develop and a rebound effect may result, with the tissues becoming even more swollen than before.

Some over-the-counter products, such as Ornade and Allerest, combine antihistamines and decongestants. The stimulant effect of the decongestant is offset by the drowsiness induced by the antihistamine.

Cortisone

If you have a severe allergy attack that cannot be controlled by antihistamines or decongestants, your doctor may prescribe a corticosteroid medication, specifically cortisone. Corticosteroids are anti-inflammatory agents, not the anabolic steroids used by some bodybuilders. They counteract the inflammation caused by allergens, as well as by non-allergic factors. They must be taken under strict medical supervision, as they have potential side effects.

Short-term use of cortisone in low doses is relatively safe, with the side effects consisting mainly of headaches, stomach upset, and fluid retention. However, prolonged use can cause:

- Elevation of blood pressure.
- Weight gain and fluid retention.
- Formation of a gastric ulcer.
- Electrolyte abnormalities.
- Psychological disorders.
- Menstrual irregularities.
- Impaired growth in children.
- Increased blood-sugar levels in diabetics.

Cortisone can be injected, taken orally, or applied topically, but it should be used only on a short-term basis due to the possibility of severe side effects. Using it topically by spraying it into your nose is much safer than taking it orally or by injection.

Inhalers containing cortisone are better than pills because the medicine can act directly on the lining of the respiratory tract, which reduces some of the side effects. While inhalers are not effective *during* acute asthma attacks, they have been found useful for preventing attacks.

Steroid inhalers do have the side effect of causing an overgrowth of the common yeast *Candida albicans,* which can lead to thrush, an infection of the mouth. Since cortisone suppresses the immune system, do not use it if you have any kind of infection. It can increase the possibility of developing a respiratory-tract infection, which is a serious problem for people with asthma.

Cromolyn

Cromolyn (Nasalchrom) was originally isolated from a plant (*Ammi visnaga*) native to the Mediterranean and was used to treat asthma by the ancient Egyptians. It will not reverse an acute asthma attack, but it can be effective at preventing attacks. It is most effective when applied locally—that is, sprayed into the nose for allergic rhinitis and inhaled from an inhaler for asthma. Side effects are extremely rare. Cromolyn is now available without a prescription.

Cromolyn works by reducing the release of histamine from the allergy-sensitive cells in the nose, helping to decrease the allergic reaction before it starts. It won't relieve your symptoms if you are in the midst of an acute attack, but if you start using it a few weeks before the allergy season begins, it may be helpful.

Bronchodilators

During an asthma attack, the air passages in the lungs become narrowed and breathing becomes difficult. Bronchodilators relax the bronchial muscles and open the airways. These medications work by stimulating the beta receptors on the cells in a way that is similar to the action of the hormone adrenaline. Some of the more common bronchodilators are:

- Albuterol (Ventolin, Proventil).
- Isoetharine (Bronkometer, Bronkosol).
- Isoproterenol (Isuprel, Medihaler-Iso).
- Pirbuterol (Maxair).
- Terbutaline (Brethine, Bricanyl).

Bronchodilators are effective at relieving acute asthma attacks, but they work only for three to six hours. If you overuse them, you *decrease* their effectiveness and *increase* the risk of such side effects as increased heart rate, elevated blood pressure, insomnia, and anxiety. In fact, Proventil and Ventolin, instead of relieving the symptoms of an asthma attack, have sometimes unexpectedly produced a life-threatening bronchial spasm.

IMMUNOTHERAPY

If neither avoidance nor medications are effective, your doctor might suggest immunotherapy, or desensitization shots, to provide relief. Immunotherapy does not cure allergies, but it can be very effective at controlling allergy symptoms. It works most effectively against dust mites, animal dander, insect stings, and grass, weed, and tree pollens. It is less effective against molds and is not particularly useful for treating food allergies. In general, it is recommended only for people with a history of severe or prolonged allergic rhinitis, or who have allergic asthma and are unable to avoid the allergen.

Immunotherapy consists of a series of injections of a solution containing the allergen. The treatment usually begins with a weak solution given once or twice a week. The strength of the solution is gradually increased, and, once the strongest dosage is reached, monthly injections are given to control the symptoms. It takes six months to a year for any improvement to be noticed. If the shots are effective, they are generally continued for three to five years, until the symptoms are gone or can be controlled with mild medication for one year. If the shots are not effective after two to three years, they are generally stopped.

Immunotherapy works by helping the body build resistance to the effects of the allergen. The concept is to stimulate the IgG antibodies to compete with the allergy-triggering IgE antibodies. The disadvantages of allergy shots, besides being time-consuming, are their expense, discomfort, and lack of guaranteed results. There is also the possibility that a shot will trigger an allergy attack or even the potentially life-threatening anaphylaxis.

Allergy shots should always be given by a medical professional, and the patient should be observed for at least thirty minutes following the shot. Harriet G. had two life-threatening episodes following shots. She had suffered from hay fever even as a child, and her doctors had convinced her mother that she would develop asthma if she was not treated. She was given shots for several years, but to little effect. "All they did," Harriet says, "was postpone the start of the season by a couple of weeks, and I still suffered until the first frost." At fourteen, after her dosage was increased, Harriet immediately developed itching and tightening of her throat, and had great difficulty breathing. Her mother rushed her back to the doctor's office, where it took three injections of epinephrine to reverse the reaction. Harriet stopped taking the allergy shots and began using Benadryl, which gave her moderate relief and made her very sleepy.

Several years later, while working in a hospital as an X-ray technician, Harriet decided to try the allergy shots again because the Benadryl was not a good solution either. If she took the Benadryl, she was too sleepy to work, but if she didn't take it, she sneezed and blew her nose so much that patients didn't want to be treated by her. Once again, when the dosage of the shots was increased, she experienced a life-threatening reaction, but this time, even after three injections of adrenaline, she didn't respond. Luckily, when she heard the doctors talking about performing a tracheotomy, "My own natural adrenaline must have kicked in, because I came out of it," she said. Needless to say, Harriet doesn't take allergy shots anymore.

EMERGENCY MEASURES

If you know you are severely allergic to insect stings and are prone to anaphylaxis, you should always carry an emergency treatment kit with you when you go out of doors. In addition, be sure you know how to use it. All of these kits contain epinephrine in an injecting device. One of the simplest devices is a spring-loaded injector that automatically administers a pre-measured dose of epinephrine when pressed against the thigh.

If you experience constriction in your throat or difficult breathing after inadvertently eating an allergy-causing food, you must be treated immediately with epinephrine. Food-induced anaphylaxis is every bit as dangerous as anaphylaxis caused by insect stings. So, if you have a history of severe reactions to certain foods, you should carry injectable epinephrine with you at all times.

Although conventional treatment can help control allergy symptoms, total avoidance, the best option, is nearly impossible, and allergy medications do have side effects. The medication side effects can range from mild, such as dryness and drowsiness, to much more serious, such as systemic reactions, including even, in the worst cases, death. In the following chapters, we will take a look at alternative natural therapies that have brought safe and effective relief to many people with allergies without harmful side effects.

3

Nutritional Therapy

Nutritionally oriented practitioners treat allergies with dietary modification and nutritional supplementation. These treatments can be used in a variety of ways. When used alone, they are considered alternative. When used in combination with other treatments, whether conventional medicine or other alternative methods, they are considered complementary. This chapter will explain how dietary modification and nutritional supplementation can bring allergy relief.

DIETARY MODIFICATION

Foods and beverages can act as drugs in the body and can be potent medicines. In fact, some of the natural active agents in food have been extracted and are used in concentrated form for therapeutic purposes. Some foods and beverages are sources of discomfort and should be avoided.

Foods and Beverages to Add

When most people think of allergies, they think first of removing foods from the diet. However, there are a number of foods that should be added to the diet to help ease or combat allergy symptoms.

Water keeps the body hydrated. Drink at least twelve glasses of pure water daily, and even more if you are physically active. The reason you need to stay hydrated is that histamine production increases if the body's water-storage level is low. The consequence of elevated histamine levels is an increase in allergic symptoms. *Barley water* relieves bronchial spasms. *Coffee* acts as a natural bronchodilator and can be useful in an emergency if your asthma medication is not available. *Grape juice* clears the lungs and soothes coughs.

Citrus rinds are a wonderful source of the bioflavonoids. You can make yourself a healthy snack, and at the same time increase your consumption of the bioflavonoids, by cooking strips of orange, lemon, and grapefruit rind in honey until soft. Another fruit that combats allergy symptoms is the *pineapple.* Pineapple helps dissolve mucus.

Hot peppers help clear sinus congestion. Fresh habaneros are the most effective, but the more readily available cayenne pepper also is effective and can easily be sprinkled on food. Capsaicin, the active ingredient in hot peppers, promotes drainage.

Horseradish also helps clear congestion. Try placing a small dish of horseradish near your bed at night to keep your nasal passages clear. You also can use horseradish as a condiment with food, or mix it with apple cider vinegar and take a quarter teaspoon four times daily. Slowly increase the amount to a half teaspoon. *Note:* If you are sensitive to mold, omit the apple cider vinegar.

Onions are a rich source of the bioflavonoid quercetin, which, in addition to having a stabilizing effect on the mast cells and basophils, has anti-inflammatory properties. Raw onion acts as an expectorant and can be used as an emergency measure when you have an asthma attack and you don't have your medication available. A slice of raw onion placed under the tongue acts as a natural bronchodilator.

Yogurt can introduce friendly bacteria into the system. If you are sensitive to dairy products, take lactobacillus capsules containing several million of that bacteria per gram.

Raw *honey* is full of pollen and can cause a natural desensitization to many different types of pollen. To help control your specific allergies, try to purchase honey from beekeepers in your local area. One tablespoon of honey mixed with one tablespoon of apple cider vinegar in a glass of water is a good beverage to drink for hay-fever relief. *Note:* If you are sensitive to mold, omit the apple cider vinegar.

Foods and Beverages to Avoid

Mucus-forming foods will increase your susceptibility to allergies because, if you have heavy mucus in your respiratory tract and an allergen becomes trapped in it, the allergen will continue to irritate your system for a longer period of time, leading to more symptoms. Dairy products and flour are mucus-forming.

Foods high in arachidonic acid, present in most animal fats, produce leukotriene cascades. Leukotriene, a substance released during allergic reactions, is up to a thousand times more potent than histamine. Shellfish and red meat are high in arachidonic acid.

Two months before the beginning of the allergy season, start to reduce your consumption of mucus-forming foods and foods high in arachidonic acid. During the allergy season, avoid them entirely.

If you are sensitive to mold, avoid foods that contain fungi or yeast, since these foods can initiate an allergic reaction. In fact, if you suspect that something in your refrigerator is spoiled, don't even smell it because if mold spores are present and you inhale them, they could set off your allergies. In addition, avoid the following foods—beer, cheese, dried fruits, fruit juice, mushrooms, pickles, soy sauce, sugar, tomato products, tofu, and vinegar.

If you have a grass allergy, you may also be allergic to sugar cane, since it is a form of grass. If you must use sugar, be sure it comes from beets or fruit. If you are allergic to ragweed, avoid eating melons because the protein responsible for allergies in ragweed also is present in melons and could cause an allergic reaction.

Dietary Suggestions

A low-protein diet helps reduce the immune system's reactivity. If you are allergic, increase your intake of fruits, vegetables, and starches, and reduce your intake of animal, dairy, and vegetable protein.

If you have chronic allergies or asthma, and prefer not to take medication, you might want to try the diet created by Michael Murray, ND. Dr. Murray's diet is rather restrictive, but it has had some remarkable results. In just four months, 72 percent of the people who followed the diet had a positive response, and the people who followed it for a year had a 92-percent response.

On Dr. Murray's diet, the following foods are allowed:

Beans (except soybeans)	Gooseberries
Beets	Herbal teas and spices
Black currants	Jerusalem artichokes
Blueberries	Lettuce
Broccoli	Nettles
Cabbage	Onions
Carrots	Pears
Cauliflower	Plums
Celery	Radishes
Cloudberries	Raspberries
Cucumbers	Strawberries

The following foods are forbidden:

Apples	Fish
Chlorinated tap water	Green peas
Chocolate	Meat
Citrus fruits	Salt
Coffee	Soybeans
Dairy products	Sugar
Eggs	Tea

In addition, with the exception of rice, millet, and buckwheat, all grains should be excluded. This is because they contain gluten, which is difficult for highly allergic people to assimilate and absorb. Rice, millet, and buckwheat do not contain gluten and can be consumed in restricted amounts.

The beneficial effects of Dr. Murray's diet are probably related to the elimination of common food allergens and to an alteration in fatty-acid metabolism. A positive side effect of the diet is that, in addition to being effective against asthma, it has been found to reduce the inclination to contract infectious diseases.

NUTRITIONAL SUPPLEMENTATION

In their search for better health, and in an attempt to avoid the side effects of medication, more and more people are using supplements. Sales of dietary supplements—including vitamins, minerals, amino acids, and herbs—are at an estimated $9.8 billion a year and growing at a rate of 10 to 12 percent annually.

Certain supplements, particularly selenium and vitamins C and E, function as antioxidants, substances that prevent damage to the cells by free radicals, or pro-oxidants. A free radical is a molecule that is missing an electron. These molecules, in an effort to balance themselves, steal electrons from other molecules. If an antioxidant is present, it may donate one of its electrons to the free radical. If there are no antioxidants present, the free radical will steal an electron from a vital cell structure. When this happens, more and more free radicals are created, causing cellular damage and leading eventually to disease.

When the mast cells are exposed to free radicals, they become fragile and more likely to release histamine and other inflammatory compounds, which increase allergy misery. Environmental sources that add to the free-radical load are cigarette smoke, air pollutants, pesticides, sunlight, fried foods, solvents, alcohol, formaldehyde, and X-rays. The following supplements, listed in their order of importance to allergy relief, are the most helpful for reducing allergy misery.

Quercetin

Quercetin is one of the bioflavonoids, a category of nutritional supplements sometimes referred to as vitamin P. The bioflavonoids act synergistically with vitamin C, which means that, when taken together, they enhance each other's effects.

The bioflavonoid quercetin is present in citrus fruits, especially in the white portion just below the skin, and in other fruits, including apples, apricots, cherries, black currants, grapes, prunes, elderberries, and rose hips. Vegetables containing quercetin are broccoli, summer squash, peppers, and onions. Quercetin also is present in the herbs chervil, hawthorn berry, horsetail, and shepherd's purse.

Unfortunately, quercetin is not present in any of the above-mentioned foods in large amounts. In fact, in order to get enough, you would need to consume so many of these fruits and vegetables that you would very likely end up with diarrhea.

BENEFITS

Quercetin actually inhibits the release of histamine and other inflammatory mediators from the mast cells, thereby reducing the allergic/inflammatory response. Antihistamines work by interfering with the binding of histamine to cells after its release. The bioflavonoids, however, prevent histamine release in the first place.

Quercetin is a potent antioxidant and inhibits the formation of inflammatory compounds such as leukotrienes, which, as previously mentioned, are a thousand times more potent in stimulating inflammatory processes than histamine. It has an effect similar to that of cromolyn, and like cromolyn, for conditions such as hay fever, it is better used as a preventive than a treatment. The downside is that, like cromolyn, quercetin is not absorbed very well. However, you can increase its efficacy by combining it with an equal amount of bromelain, an anti-inflammatory enzyme from the pineapple plant that increases the absorption and tissue concentration of a variety of compounds and also may increase the absorption of quercetin.

Quercetin also protects the arteries and helps prevent cancer.

DOSAGE

Take 250 to 500 milligrams of quercetin ten minutes before meals.

Start taking quercetin at least two weeks before the hay fever season begins and continue taking it until the end of the season.

SIDE EFFECTS

Although quercetin is non-toxic, it should not be taken by pregnant women, according to Andrew Weil, MD, an author and lecturer who teaches about alternative medicine and mind-body interaction at the Program in Integrative Medicine at the College of Medicine, University of Arizona.

Extremely high doses of quercetin may cause diarrhea, but this side effect is more likely to result when consuming food sources of the nutrient, since they are needed in such large amounts.

Bee Pollen

Bee pollen is the powdery material gathered by bees from the stamens of flowering plants. It contains several nutrients, including the B-complex vitamins, vitamin C, and beta-carotene, in addition to the minerals calcium, copper, iron, magnesium, potassium, manganese, and sodium. It also is a rich source of the essential fatty acids and enzymes.

Bee pollen strengthens the immune system. In addition, it functions like desensitization shots against allergies caused by pollen.

Bee pollen is the only substance in the world that contains all the enzymes, hormones, vitamins, and amino acids that the body needs. It is also useful for treating digestive upsets, prostate problems, acne, fatigue, sore throat, and sexual problems.

DOSAGE

Use raw crude pollen produced within ten miles of your home, if possible. Start with a few granules at a time and gradually work up to two teaspoons daily. Bee pollen works best when taken on an empty stomach. Note that its effect most likely will not be instantaneous, but rather progressive. However, you should notice improvement within about a month.

SIDE EFFECTS

Bee pollen can cause an allergic reaction in some people. Do not use it if it causes any discomfort, such as a rash or wheezing.

Vitamin C

Vitamin C is an antioxidant that is required for collagen formation, tissue growth, and tissue repair. So many foods are rich sources of vitamin C that you would think you could obtain enough through the diet. However, since it is a water-soluble nutrient, most of it is either destroyed in cooking or excreted in the urine. In addition, if you smoke, note that cigarettes destroy from 25 to 100 milligrams of vitamin C each!

The following fruits are good sources of vitamin C—avocados, black currants, cantaloupe, grapefruit, lemons, mangoes, oranges, papayas, persimmons, pineapple, rose hips, and strawberries.

Vegetables that contain vitamin C include asparagus, beet greens, broccoli, Brussels sprouts, collards, dandelion greens, dulse, kale, mustard greens, onions, green peas, sweet peppers, radishes, Swiss chard, tomatoes, turnip greens, and watercress.

Vitamin C also is present in the herbs alfalfa, burdock root, cayenne, chickweed, eyebright, fennel seed, fenugreek, hops, horsetail, kelp, peppermint, parsley, pine needle, plantain, raspberry leaf, red clover, skullcap, violet leaves, yarrow, and yellow dock.

BENEFITS

Vitamin C is an antioxidant. It prevents the secretion of histamine by the white blood cells, increases the detoxification of histamine, and lowers the blood-histamine levels. It also inhibits bronchial constriction in both normal and asthmatic subjects.

In addition, vitamin C helps heal wounds and burns, aids in preventing many bacterial and viral infections, helps counteract the formation of some cancer-causing substances, and is useful in preventing and healing colds.

DOSAGE

In a study at the Food and Nutrition Laboratory of Arizona State University in Tempe, people with hay fever who were given 2,000 milligrams of vitamin C daily had their histamine production drop by 38 percent. Most practitioners recommend 500 to 1,000 milligrams of vitamin C three to four times daily for treating allergies. Vitamin C is harmless and can be taken to bowel tolerance, which is the amount that causes diarrhea. Simply cut back the dose until the diarrhea subsides.

Large amounts of vitamin C have been known to cause the formation of uric-acid stones and to reverse the anticoagulant activity of the drug coumadin. If you are diabetic, your medication may need to be adjusted.

Vitamin E

Vitamin E is a fat-soluble antioxidant composed of compounds called tocopherols. It protects other fat-soluble vitamins from being destroyed by oxygen.

The best sources of vitamin E are cold-pressed vegetable oils, organ meats, and eggs. Vitamin E also is present in leafy green vegetables, legumes, nuts, seeds, broccoli, Brussels sprouts, soybeans, wheat germ, and whole grains.

If you are on a low-fat diet, you are probably not getting enough vitamin E from food sources. In addition, whether or not you are vegetarian, 60 to 70 percent of the vitamin E you consume is excreted in the feces.

BENEFITS

Vitamin E is a powerful antioxidant. It aids immune function, lowers histamine production, and helps protect the lungs against air pollution.

Vitamin E also accelerates healing, eases leg cramps, helps prevent and dissolve blood clots, and alleviates fatigue. It can help maintain a youthful appearance by retarding cellular aging due to oxidation.

DOSAGE

Take 600 to 800 international units of vitamin E daily in divided doses. It is best to begin by taking it in a low dose and then build up to the recommended dose slowly, as vitamin E sometimes has a tendency to raise the blood pressure.

SIDE EFFECTS

If you are allergic to wheat or soy, do not take natural vitamin E, which is derived from these products. Instead, use dry vitamin E acetate or succinate, and take twice as much, since the dry form is only half as potent.

It you have an overactive thyroid, diabetes, high blood pressure, or rheumatic heart disease, it is extremely important to start with a very low dose and build up gradually. A good method is to start with 100 international units daily for a month, then take 200 international units for another month, and so on, until you reach the optimum dose. If you have any of the aforementioned conditions, take vitamin E under a doctor's supervision.

Selenium

Selenium is an antioxidant that is absorbed by plants from the soil. The amount of selenium that is present in a food depends on how much was in the particular soil in which the food was grown. Unfortunately, the continued application of chemical fertilizers has removed a good deal of selenium from the soil. Furthermore, processed foods are very low in selenium.

Some selenium is present in meat, chicken, seafood, salmon, and dairy products. It also can be found in grains, wheat germ, Brazil nuts, brewer's yeast, broccoli, brown rice, garlic, molasses, onions, and tomatoes.

BENEFITS

Selenium helps decrease sensitivity to airborne allergens. It works synergistically with vitamin E, which means that when selenium and vitamin E are taken together, they increase each other's ability to protect the body.

Selenium also helps maintain elasticity in the tissues, relieves menopausal symptoms, and provides protection against some cancers.

DOSAGE
Take 100 to 200 micrograms of selenium daily.

SIDE EFFECTS
To date, no side effects have been recorded for selenium. In fact, Dr. Edward M. Wagner, a Philadelphia-based nutritionist, notes that several years ago 30,000 micrograms were mistakenly included in a multivitamin, and although this is a very large amount, no adverse effects were reported.

The B Vitamins
The B vitamins are involved in the body's energy production. They are water soluble and not stored in the body. They are synergistic, which means they work together to help maintain health. Although all of the B vitamins are essential, the three that are the most helpful for allergy relief are vitamins B_5, B_6, and B_{12}. Following are sources, benefits, dosages, and side effects of these three nutrients.

Vitamin B_5

Vitamin B_5, also known as pantothene, is found in beef, pork, organ meats, saltwater fish, and eggs. It is also present in uncooked vegetables, brewer's yeast, and whole grains.

BENEFITS

Vitamin B_5 stimulates the adrenal glands to produce cortisone, which helps counteract the inflammation caused by allergens. It also helps the body utilize other vitamins, enhances stamina, and helps the digestive tract function normally.

DOSAGE

Take 500 milligrams of vitamin B_5 twice daily.

SIDE EFFECTS

Vitamin B_5 has no appreciable side effects or contraindications.

Vitamin B_6

Some vitamin B_6 is present in most foods. The best sources are beef, organ meats, eggs, milk, brewer's yeast, wheat bran and wheat germ, cantaloupe, cabbage, and blackstrap molasses.

BENEFITS

Vitamin B_6 acts as an antihistamine and reduces the severity of symptoms related to airborne allergies. It also has been shown to reduce the frequency and severity of wheezing and asthma attacks.

Vitamin B_6 also aids fat and protein metabolism, and helps maintain a proper electrolyte balance. It has a mild diuretic effect that helps reduce the symptoms of premenstrual syndrome. Vitamin B_6 helps protect the heart, supports the nervous and immune systems, and aids vitamin-B_{12} absorption.

DOSAGE

Take 250 milligrams of vitamin B_6 three times daily.

Do not take vitamin B_6 if you are using L-dopa to treat Parkinson's disease.

Vitamin B$_{12}$

Vitamin B_{12} is available primarily from animal sources, such as beef, pork, organ meats, seafood, eggs, milk, and cheese. If you are a vegetarian, you do not get enough vitamin B_{12} from your food unless you eat lots of sea vegetables and soybeans, the only vegetable foods in which it is found. The herbs alfalfa, bladderwort, and hops also contain some B_{12}.

BENEFITS

Taking vitamin B_{12} has resulted in definite improvement in asthma patients. People with asthma who received weekly intramuscular injections of 1,000 micrograms had less shortness of breath during exercise, as well as improved appetite, sleep, and general health.

Vitamin B_{12} works synergistically with the other B vitamins and with vitamins A, C, and E. It is necessary for the prevention of anemia and works with other nutrients to help the body utilize iron and form red blood cells. It also aids the absorption and metabolism of food, keeps the cells healthy, prevents nerve damage, and enhances memory.

DOSAGE

About 1 to 3 milligrams of vitamin B_{12} taken orally may provide benefits similar to those of the injectable form. Some nutritionists recommend taking vitamin B_{12} in the sublingual form for better absorption.

Always take a vitamin-B complex when you take a high dose of any single B vitamin because megadoses of one taken over a long period of time may cause deficiencies in the others. The B vitamins work more effectively when taken all together.

Beta-carotene

Beta-carotene is the best known of the carotenoids, a class of compounds related to vitamin A. When you eat foods containing beta-carotene or take beta-carotene supplements, the nutrient is converted to vitamin A in your liver. Large amounts of vitamin A can be toxic to your liver, but beta-carotene is not toxic because the body utilizes only what it needs, eliminating the rest.

The best sources of beta-carotene are fish liver oil, eggs, dairy products, and green and yellow fruits and vegetables. Herbs that contain beta-carotene include alfalfa, borage leaves, burdock root, cayenne, chickweed, eyebright, fennel seed, hops, horsetail, lemongrass, mullein, nettle, oat straw, paprika, parsley, peppermint, plantain, raspberry leaf, red clover, rose hips, sage, violet leaves, and watercress.

BENEFITS

Beta-carotene increases the integrity of the mucous membrane of the respiratory tract and decreases leukotriene formation.

Beta-carotene also helps prevent eye problems and skin disorders, acts as an antioxidant, boosts the immune system, helps protect the cells against cancer, and slows the aging process.

DOSAGE

Take 30,000 to 50,000 international units of beta-carotene twice daily.

If you have diabetes or an underactive thyroid, avoid beta-carotene because your system cannot convert it to vitamin A.

You cannot overdose on beta-carotene, but if you take too much, your skin may turn yellowish orange.

Magnesium

Magnesium is known as the healthy heart mineral. It is vital for the body's production of energy and necessary for the proper utilization of calcium and potassium.

Magnesium is present in most foods and is especially abundant in meat, fish and seafood, and dairy products. It is also present in many fruits, such as apples, bananas, figs, grapefruit, and peaches. In addition, magnesium can be found in yellow corn, avocados, dark green vegetables, almonds and other nuts, seeds, wheat products, and whole grains.

BENEFITS

Magnesium is an essential mineral for nerve and muscle function and enzyme activity. It keeps histamine levels in check and relaxes the smooth muscles of the bronchioles.

Magnesium also helps prevent depression, heart disease, and high blood pressure. It aids in bone formation and mineral metabolism.

DOSAGE

Take 1,000 milligrams of magnesium daily in divided doses. If you take a multivitamin, check to see if it contains magnesium. If it does, subtract the amount it contains from 1,000 milligams and take the remaining amount.

 Magnesium may have a laxative effect, so if you suffer diarrhea, cut back the dosage. If you have diseased kidneys, do not take more than 300 milligrams of magnesium daily.

Buying Nutritional Supplements

Buying nutritional supplements can be confusing, not only because they come in so many different forms and strengths, but also because so many different brands are available.

You will usually find higher-quality supplements in health food stores than in supermarkets and chain drug stores. In addition, if you have any questions, you are more likely to get knowledgeable help in a health food store.

Supplements are available in a variety of forms. They come as liquids, capsules, caplets, tablets, and powders. Liquids enter the system faster than the other forms. Capsules contain liquid or powder, and are usually easier to swallow than tablets. Caplets look like capsules, but are really tablets. A tablet is a molded block of solid material whose contents can be designed to be absorbed quickly or slowly. Powders have to be mixed with some form of liquid and are useful if you have to take a large amount of a particular nutrient.

Supplements contain dosages of the nutrients that are much higher than the recommended daily allowances (RDAs). The RDAs are the federal government's nutritional standards, designed to prevent diseases that result from deficiencies, such as scurvy and beriberi. However, the dosages are not adequate for good health. Scientific studies have shown that our bodies work better when we take larger doses of the nutrients.

Supplements may contain one or a number of nutrients, and

these are listed on the label. Every label should give a complete list of the ingredients, the recommended dosage, and directions for taking the supplement.

Safety of Nutritional Supplements

Taking megadoses of individual supplements over long periods of time may cause deficiencies in the body's supply of other nutrients and also may have an effect on any medications you may be taking. Be sure to tell your healthcare practitioner if you are using any supplements in megadose amounts.

PREVENTION OF FOOD ALLERGIES

Dr. Edward M. Wagner believes that when food is not digested properly, the immune system identifies it as a foreign object and tries to defend the body against it. He suggests that people with allergies take digestive enzymes with their meals to break food down into the smallest possible molecules. He also believes that one cause of food allergies, especially among the elderly, is repetitive dining. Eating the same foods day after day can cause sensitivities that can lead to food allergies.

The *rotation diet* is a simple yet effective method for preventing problems with food allergies. If you rotate the foods you eat every four days, you will not eat any one food more often than once in every four days.

If you are considering self-testing for food allergies, you may want to try the following natural method. For three days, eat nothing but brown rice and clarified butter. This will clear out all the undigested food from your body. On the fourth day, begin adding one food at a time, at least three hours apart. This way, if you have an allergic reaction, you will be able to tell which food is the culprit.

Nutritional therapy for treating allergies is inexpensive, has no side effects, and benefits approximately 75 percent of the people who follow the recommended diet and take the supplements. However, if you take medication for asthma or any acute form of allergic reaction, do not stop taking it too abruptly. Try to find a nutritionally oriented practitioner who will monitor your progress and wean you off your medication slowly.

4

Herbal Therapy

Humans have used herbal remedies to treat illness for thousands of years, and many people throughout the world still use herbs because they are safe, reliable, and have no side effects. Currently, about 50 million Americans use botanical supplements. Herbal remedies do not provide the quick fix of most of the traditional allergy medications, but while traditional allergy drugs may relieve the symptoms, they don't help heal the underlying problems that cause the allergies. Herbal remedies *do*. Herbs may have to be used daily for long periods of time, sometimes for several weeks, but they do help the body return to its natural state of well-being.

A SHORT HISTORY OF HERBAL THERAPY

Medicinal herbal remedies have been used throughout history. During the third millennium B.C., doctors in ancient China compiled manuals, known as herbals, that depicted the plants used for medicinal purposes. A Chinese text written about 2700 B.C. lists thirteen herbal prescriptions.

In ancient Egypt, the *Papyrus Ebers,* written in 1500 B.C., contained references to more than 700 herbal remedies. In ancient Greece, Hippocrates, known as the Father of Medicine, often used diet and herbs as the basis of his treatments. In the latter part of the first century A.D., Greek physician and pharmacologist Pedanius Dioscorides compiled *De materia medica,* an herbal treatise describing approximately 1,000 drugs and remedies. First published in A.D. 77 and translated into several languages, it was the foremost authority on botany and pharmacology in the West for the next 1,500 years. Herbs also were used extensively in the Roman Empire.

Herbal remedies were used for centuries, until World War II, when the new synthetic drugs came on the market and began their supreme reign, especially in the United States. However, as people have become more concerned about the side effects of conventional drugs, herbal medicine has once again gained in popularity because herbs are considered a safer alternative, with fewer side effects. Furthermore, when people use herbal remedies, they feel they are maintaining some control over their health.

BENEFITS OF HERBS

Herbs have a cleansing effect, help normalize body function, and help nourish the body as well as alleviate allergies. Herbs raise the body's energy level, and stimulate and strengthen the body's immune system. Herbs encourage the body's natural healing mechanism, and many herbs contain compounds such as the bioflavanoids that help prevent the formation of histamine.

Herbal remedies can be gentle, effective, and inexpensive alternatives to conventional allergy medications. They can be used in conjunction with traditional medicine and as complements to other treatments. They are natural remedies, known to be safer and to have fewer side effects than drugs. Herbal therapy, as part of a holistic healing program that also addresses diet and lifestyle, works to eliminate the causes of symptoms, rather than just temporarily suppress them.

HERBS THAT TREAT ALLERGIES

Many herbs and combinations of herbs can help provide relief from various types of allergies. The herbs discussed in the following pages are the ones most often recommended. Note that in the following descriptions, when a dosage is not given, it is because the strength of the preparation may vary and the amount suggested on the label of the particular product should be used. (For directions on preparing teas, decoctions, and other forms recommended for taking herbs, see "Preparing Herbs" on page 68.)

Herbs for the Respiratory Tract

In addition to strengthening the respiratory tract, the following herbs help alleviate congestion and inflammation, promote drainage, and encourage mucus to be expelled from the lungs:

- *Angelica* inhibits the production of IgE antibodies. For best results, drink three cups of angelica tea every day.
- *Bayberry* reduces secretions. To alleviate congestion, use it as a gargle or as a compress on your chest.
- *Cayenne* has, as its active ingredient, capsaicin, which helps promote drainage in the respiratory system. Cayenne is inexpensive and readily available. James Braly, MD, medical director of Immuno Labs in Fort Lauderdale, Florida, recommends cayenne pepper to his allergy patients. These patients have reversed their allergies simply by sprinkling large amounts of cayenne pepper on their food. In some patients, the conditions even reversed overnight.

  One of Dr. Braly's patients had suffered from such severe nightly asthma attacks that it was impossible for him to lie down without coughing or wheezing. He had to sit upright all night, which made it extremely difficult to sleep. The man reported to Dr. Braly that after the first day of using cayenne on his food, he had found himself symptom-free for the first time in thirteen years.
- *Elder* helps ease congestion and inflammation.
- *Ephedra* relieves nasal and chest congestion. Its alkaloids are ephedrine and pseudoephedrine, both of which are bronchodilators.

  Asian ephedra (ma huang) has been used in China for more than 5,000 years for the treatment of respiratory-system problems, and, even today, various species of Asian ephedra are used as sources of both ephedrine and pseudo-ephedrine. Ephedrine is used to treat allergies and asthma because of its ability to reduce allergic reactions in the nasal cells and to relax the airways in the lungs. It was the first ma huang alkaloid to find wide use in traditional medicine. It does have the side effect of stimulating the sympathetic nervous system, which can lead to elevated blood pressure, but when the whole ephedra plant is used, and not just the isolated active ingredient, the blood pressure is not elevated as much.

Pseudoephedrine, another one of the alkaloids in ma huang, reduces the heart rate and lowers the blood pressure very slightly, thus counteracting the side effects of ephedrine. In addition, it is an effective bronchodilator, equal in strength to ephedrine, but without the side effects of heart palpitations and other cardiovascular symptoms. The decongestant Sudafed contains a chemical modeled after a constituent of ephedra.

The recommended dose of ephedra depends on the alkaloid content of the particular form used. For treating asthma, the dose should have an ephedrine content of 12.5 to 25.0 milligrams and should be taken two to three times daily. For the whole herb, the recommended dose is 500 to 1,000 milligrams three times a day. Since ephedra is such a powerful herb and its strength is often difficult to accurately determine, it is better and safer to use it in the form of a standardized preparation because its therapeutic activity will be more dependable. If you choose a form that is not standardized, start with a low dose and gradually increase to the maximum level you can tolerate.

Ephedra is quite safe when used properly. However, its

therapeutic effect may become diminished when it is used for a long period of time because ephedrine can weaken the adrenal glands. Therefore, always use ephedra along with nutrients that support the adrenal glands, such as vitamins B$_5$, B$_6$, and C, magnesium, and zinc. It is also helpful to use it in combination with herbal expectorants, such as lobelia (*Lobelia inflata*), licorice (*Glycyrrhiza glabra*), and grindelia (*Grindelia camporum*).

Check with an herbalist or nutritionally oriented healthcare practitioner before using ephedra, as it is a strong central-nervous-system stimulant. Furthermore, *do not* use ephedra if you are taking a monoamine oxidase (MAO) inhibitor or if you have high blood pressure, diabetes, a heart disorder, a thyroid problem, or glaucoma.

- *Eucalyptus* helps clear mucus from the nose and lungs, and relieves upper-respiratory distress. Use it in the form of lozenges, an ointment, or a liquid, or steep the leaves in boiling water and inhale the vapors.
- *Eyebright* contains flavonoids that are anti-inflammatory and stabilize the mast cells that line the nasal passages. Take eyebright according to the directions on the bottle.
- *Fenugreek* helps break up mucus in the respiratory tract. Drink two cups of fenugreek tea daily.
- *Feverfew* enhances fatty-acid metabolism and significantly reduces arachidonic-acid formation. This reduces histamine and leukotriene production.
- *Fritillary,* a Chinese herb that is related to the lily, makes an effective cough syrup when combined with Chinese loquat fruit and licorice root.
- *Garlic* lowers the IgE-antibody count. It can be taken in fresh form or tablet form.

- *Ginger,* in tea form, has decongestant properties. Drink the tea and inhale the vapors.
- *Ginkgo biloba* is an antioxidant and expectorant that aids in expelling mucus from the lungs.
- *Goldenrod* helps eliminate mucus. Drink the tea and inhale the vapors.
- *Goldenseal* helps eliminate mucus and aids in the absorption of nutrients. *Do not* take goldenseal if you are allergic to ragweed. In addition, *do not* take goldenseal daily for more than one week at a time.
- *Lemongrass* has decongestant properties. Drink the tea and inhale the vapors.
- *Mullein,* in tea form, is useful for treating hay fever. Drink two cups of tea daily.
- *Myrrh* is an astringent that helps control inflammation and reduces secretions and discharges. Take it as directed on the label.
- *Red sage* helps eliminate mucus. Take it as directed on the label.
- *Reishi,* a mushroom, reduces histamine release, relaxes the respiratory tract, enhances fatty-acid metabolism, and decreases the amount of leukotrienes. It is available in gourmet food stores and is a delicious addition to recipes. It is also available at health food stores as tablets and capsules.
- *Rosemary* has decongestant properties. Drink the tea and inhale the vapors.
- *Sage* has decongestant properties. Drink the tea and inhale the vapors.
- *Squill* is useful for treating bronchial asthma accompanied by a dry irritable cough due to decreased sputum production. It makes mucous secretions more fluid and easier to expectorate. Take it as directed on the label.

- *Stinging nettle* can be used as a preventive beginning two to three weeks before the start of hay-fever season. It can also lessen allergy symptoms after the season has started. Recommended by herbalists since the tenth century A.D., it effectively relieves allergies when used as an extract made from the fresh, undried plant.

  A February 1990 study reported in the *Journal of Medicinal Plant Research* showed that freeze-dried stinging nettle relieved allergy symptoms in more than half of the participating patients. Stinging nettle is non-toxic, is a good source of trace minerals, and has a long history of use as an edible green and an herbal tea. Many of the patients who suffered from hay fever were able to stop using antihistamines.

  One or two 300-milligram capsules of freeze-dried stinging nettle taken twice daily can help control or prevent allergy symptoms during hay-fever season. Because it is non-toxic, it can even be taken every two to four hours. Note, however, that stinging nettle does have a slight diuretic effect.
- *Yerba maté,* in tea form, helps relieve allergic symptoms. Place two to three teaspoons of dried herb in a pint of hot water and drink the tea on an empty stomach.
- *Yarrow* has decongestant and astringent properties that help control inflamed tissues and reduce secretions and discharges. Drink the tea and inhale the vapors.

Many people have reported that after using these herbal remedies, they were able to stop taking their prescription medications. However, it is always a good idea to tell your healthcare provider that you are using an herbal remedy. In addition, never stop taking any medication, especially one for asthma, too abruptly.

Herbs for the Skin

The following herbs are effective at soothing the skin, relieving itching, and treating a variety of allergy-related problems:

- *Black currant oil* is an excellent anti-inflammatory agent.
- *Black walnut* can be used both internally and externally to treat eczema.
- *Burdock,* in a commercially prepared form, can be applied externally to treat eczema, rashes, and hives. However, *do not* use the plant in its natural form, as it has been known to cause contact dermatitis.
- *Calendula,* which is derived from pot marigolds, soothes dry cracked skin when used as an herbal cream.
- *Chickweed,* added to bath water, will relieve itching. Use one to two cups of chickweed tea to a tub of water.
- *Evening primrose,* in oil form, softens dry, scaly, itchy skin. Massage it gently into the affected area.
- *Goldenseal* aids in treating eczema. Take it according to the directions on the bottle. Note that goldenseal is not intended for long-term use, since it can interfere with the beneficial bacteria and flora in the colon.
- *Oregon grape,* in tea form, is useful for treating eczema. You also can make a compress from the tea and apply it to the affected area.
- *Red clover* purifies the blood and soothes the nerves. Take it according to the directions on the bottle.
- *Yellow dock* has a cleansing effect on the system. However, it should not be taken in large amounts, as it can cause diarrhea.

Anything applied to the skin can be absorbed into the system. However, herbal remedies have a higher safety factor than do most medications.

PREPARING HERBS

Herbal remedies can be obtained commercially or prepared at home. Some ways to prepare them are as follows:

- *Tea.* To make one cup of tea, steep one to two tablespoons of plant parts in one cup of boiling water. Drink one cup of tea three times a day.
- *Infusion.* Similar to tea. Pour one pint of boiling water over one-half to one ounce of plant parts, and steep for ten minutes.
- *Decoction.* Simmer one-half ounce of plant parts in one cup of water for twenty to thirty minutes.
- *Cold extract.* Add one to two ounces of plant parts to a pint of cold water and allow the mixture to stand for twelve hours.
- *Tincture.* Combine four ounces of powdered or finely cut herb with one pint of brandy, vodka, or gin. Cover tightly, and shake several times daily for two weeks. Strain the liquid before using it.

In true herbalism, the essential ingredients are not separated out of the plant. When you use the whole plant, you generally do not suffer side effects, as you might when using isolated ingredients from the plant.

AYURVEDIC HERBALISM

Ayurveda is an ancient Indian healing system teaching that you should participate actively in maintaining your body system. It focuses on how to prevent disease and how to return to good health. Its two main principles are that the mind influences the physical body, and that body type has to be taken into consideration when designing a treatment plan.

Ayurvedic physicians view allergies as a result of impaired digestion. They believe that the digestive system is linked to all allergies, not just those caused by food. If a body's digestion is impaired, it has to deal with more than the average amount of toxins and eventually becomes overwhelmed and more susceptible to allergies. Ayurvedic practitioners feel that, to stimulate digestion and help the body clear out toxins, it is necessary to enhance the body's production of secretory IgA, an immune antibody common to the mucous membranes of the gastrointestinal tract.

Virender Sodhi, MD, ND, an ayurvedic practitioner from Bellevue, Washington, suggests that people with allergies take the following herbs a half-hour before meals to help produce more IgA and to stimulate digestion—black pepper, cayenne pepper, garlic, ginger, long pepper, and onion.

Dr. Sodhi also recommends taking an herbal blend called triphala three times a day in tablet form, either before or after a meal. Triphala is a combination of the East Indian herbs *chebula, chebula belerica, embilica officinalis,* and *terminalia.* Triphala can be used as both a treatment and a preventive. It aids digestion, helps eliminate toxins, and helps maintain a healthy intestinal tract.

.   .   .

Mainstream doctors are concerned that herbs may interact with each other and with other medications. At the same time, many patients don't tell their doctors if they are using herbal remedies, either because they fear their doctor's reaction or because they don't think it's important for the doctor to know. Even though most herbal remedies are non-toxic, it is a good idea—especially when the patient is a pregnant woman, child, or senior citizen—to consult with a naturopath or trained herbalist before using them.

Herbal therapy is rapidly becoming more than just a useful adjunct for treating allergies. Although orthodox medical practitioners have been reluctant to become involved with herbal remedies, nobody denies that most of the world relies on herbal therapy as the major form of healthcare. In fact, the World Health Organization has taken steps toward the worldwide promotion and support of herbal therapy in an effort to make effective, affordable healthcare available to everyone.

5

Aromatherapy

romatherapy, the use of essential oils from plants, is a branch of alternative medicine that can be considered a subspecialty of herbal therapy. Essential oils are condensed from the parts of plants that give them fragrance, protect them from predators, and attract insects for pollination. Some experts believe that essential oils carry the plant's vital energy, which in turn raises the vital energy of the person using the product. However this is achieved, essential oils do help balance the body's functioning and alleviate some medical conditions.

The principles of aromatherapy are based on folk practices,

but a number of them are being confirmed by science. Researchers have documented that tea tree oil kills bacteria, clove oil kills the tuberculosis virus, and nutmeg oil lowers the systolic blood pressure. Certain essential oils have been shown in French studies to have antibiotic and antiviral properties. Others are known to inhibit bacterial growth and to act as effective fungicides. Overall, essential oils can stimulate the body's immune system to develop natural antibodies.

Essential oils can be inhaled directly, put into boiling water for steam inhalation, or applied to the skin. Although scientists are not sure how scent affects the brain, most believe it causes a chemical and/or psychological reaction. Essential oils also can affect mood and behavior.

Courses in aromatherapy are taught in many schools, but at the present time, there are no standards in the United States for training or certification.

A SHORT HISTORY OF AROMATHERAPY

Many of the so-called alternative therapies, including aromatherapy, are based on ancient medical systems and represent a return to nature. Herbal therapy and aromatherapy are much older forms of treatment than Western orthodox medicine.

Aromatherapy was first used in the West about seventy-five years ago. A French fragrance chemist, René-Maurice Gattefosse, burned his arm while on the job and immediately plunged it into a nearby container of lavender oil. His pain eased immediately, the burn healed quickly and with little discomfort, and there was no scarring, all positive results that he attributed to lavender oil's antiseptic and anti-inflammatory properties, as well as to its potent scent. Following this experience, Gattefosse devoted his life to the study of essential oils.

French medical students were, and still are, taught how to prescribe essential oils. By the 1970s, the use of aromatherapy had grown widely in Europe and Japan, and today, aromatherapy prescriptions are covered by insurance in many European countries.

Aromatherapy is now becoming popular in the United States, but it was a different scenario fifty years ago, when the new wonder drugs first arrived on the scene. At that time, herbs and essential oils were frowned upon, even banned in some places, because they were viewed as archaic and outmoded in comparison to the wonder drugs. In fact, in 1941, the British Pharmacy and Medicine Act made the practice of herbal therapy illegal. Now, it has come full circle, and the scientific world is taking a new look at the value of natural remedies, since synthetic drugs have too many unwanted side effects and may not be as wonderful as previously supposed.

HOW AROMATHERAPY WORKS

Aromatherapy works by both inhalation and absorption. Essential oils release a gaseous vapor into the air that, when inhaled, is absorbed into the bloodstream through the lungs and the olfactory nerve, which is connected to the sense of smell. When used in bath water or added to massage oils, they are absorbed into the bloodstream through the skin and carried to the muscles, joints, tissues, and organs.

Inhalation

Aromatherapy treats the mind and body together. At the same time an oil has a chemical effect on the body, its scent has a powerful effect on the emotions.

Different scents act upon different glands and work with the endocrine system to balance and stabilize the body. Although it is focused upon less than the other senses, the sense of smell is one of our most acute senses. When a scent is inhaled, the odor molecules in the scent strike nerves in the nasal passages and are transformed into nerve impulses. These impulses then travel to the olfactory bulbs in the brain, which are directly connected to the limbic system (also known as the primitive brain), that portion of the brain that controls memory and emotion. The scent information is then passed to the hypothalamus, the part of the brain that controls the pituitary gland, which in turn responds by releasing hormones that are essential for most of the basic body functions.

There are four different inhalation techniques currently used in aromatherapy:

1. Put a few drops of an essential oil in a bowl of hot water and place the bowl near a source of heat, such as a radiator or heating vent.
2. Put five drops of a decongestant oil in a bowl of steaming water, drape a towel over your head, and inhale the vapors for three or four minutes. Keep your eyes closed.
3. Sprinkle a few drops of an expectorant oil on your pillowcase.
4. Put some essential oil on a tissue and carry the tissue in a resealable plastic bag.

Some essential oils are adaptogens, which means they have a regulating effect. The same oil—lavender, for example—can act as a sedative or a stimulant, depending on the body's need at the time.

When employing essential oils, it is important to use them in their pure form. Even though synthetic fragrances may smell just like essential oils, they do not have the same therapeutic effects.

Absorption

During an aromatherapy massage treatment, the pleasantly scented oil rubbed into the skin is absorbed into the bloodstream and has positive effects on the nervous, immune, and endocrine systems. Essential oils and massage have a synergistic effect on the body due to the interaction of touch and smell.

Using essential oils on a regular basis increases the body's resistance to illness. It also promotes a positive mental state, which helps stimulate the immune system.

Because they are so highly concentrated, full-strength essential oils can cause irritation and should not be applied directly to the skin. Dilute them in a carrier oil such as sweet almond or apricot kernel oil, the two most frequently used oils. A carrier oil is a natural medium in which the essence can be diluted without alteration of its therapeutic effects.

Two essential oils can be applied full strength to the skin, however. Lavender oil helps the skin heal and can be applied directly to insect bites, rashes, and even burns and cuts. Tea tree oil is also non-irritating and has been touted as a "first-aid kit in a bottle." It has anti-infectious, anti-inflammatory, antiseptic, antiviral, and antifungal properties.

ESSENTIAL OILS THAT TREAT ALLERGIES

Essential oils, like herbs, are best used in their whole, natural form. If the active ingredient in an oil is extracted and used alone, it is less effective. Unlike medications, which usually contain only a single molecule, aromatic oils contain several molecules, in different proportions, that all reinforce each other. You can, though, very effectively mix oils together to create a synergistic blend.

Following are some essential oils and oil combinations that you might wish to try to help alleviate various types of allergies.

For Allergic Congestion

EUCALYPTUS OIL

Eucalyptus has both decongestant and antiseptic properties. Put two drops on a tissue and inhale the vapors. Put five to ten drops in a vaporizer. Put five drops in a basin of hot water, drape a towel over your head, lean over the basin, and inhale the vapors. If desired, add a drop or two of blue gum oil and/or peppermint oil.

SANDALWOOD OIL

Add five drops of sandalwood oil to a small bowl of water. Place the bowl on your night table so that you can inhale the vapors while you sleep. *Note:* Keep sandalwood oil out of the reach of children and pets.

SANDALWOOD-PINE-LAVENDER OIL BLEND

Combine fifteen drops of sandalwood oil, fifteen drops of pine oil, and ten drops of lavender oil. Bring a large pot of water to a boil, then remove it from the heat and add a teaspoon of the oil blend. Drape a towel over your head, lean over the pot, and inhale the vapors for ten minutes. When finished, stay in a warm room for another thirty minutes. *Note:* If you have epilepsy or a nerve disorder, omit the pine oil.

For Allergic Skin Conditions

For most allergic skin conditions, use chamomile, melissa, tea tree, or lavender oil. First, do a patch test. Put a few drops of the oil on the back of your wrist, cover the area with a bandage, and check for redness or irritation after one hour. If no irritation occurs, apply a thin film of the oil to the affected area two to three times a day.

For Asthma

Put two drops of one, or one drop each of two or three, of the following oils on a tissue and inhale the vapors:

Benzoin oil	**Lavender oil**
Chamomile oil	**Melissa oil**
Clary sage oil	**Rose oil**
Cypress oil	**Sandalwood oil**
Frankincense oil	**Sweet marjoram oil**
Hyssop oil	**Valerian oil**

Keep the tissue in a re-sealable plastic bag and carry it with you to use when needed. *Note:* While these oils can relieve asthma symptoms and may even help prevent a full-blown attack, they are not a substitute for urgent medical treatment.

For Eczema

Add one to two drops of each of the following appropriate oils to one ounce of rose water, which is available at most pharmacies:

• For infected eczema—lavender oil, tea tree oil.

• For inflamed eczema—chamomile oil, yarrow oil.

• For scaly eczema—melissa oil, rose oil.

• For weepy eczema—myrrh oil, patchouli oil.

Dip a cloth in the solution and use it as a compress on the affected area.

For scalp eczema, add two to six drops of lavender oil or tea tree oil to one tablespoon of olive oil and rub the mixture into your scalp. Leave it on your hair for about ten minutes, then shampoo.

For Hay Fever

CHAMOMILE-LEMON OIL BLEND

Put one drop of chamomile oil and one drop of lemon oil on a tissue and inhale the vapors. If you need more relief, add a drop of peppermint oil, clove oil, rosemary oil, lavender oil, and/or geranium oil in any combination that works for you.

MAKE YOUR OWN BLEND

Combine two or three of the following oils:

Basil oil	Marjoram oil
Blue gum oil	Melissa oil
Cajeput oil	Myrtle oil
Clary sage oil	Peppermint oil
Clove oil	Pine oil
Eucalyptus oil	Rose oil
Hyssop oil	Rosemary oil
Lavender oil	Spanish sage oil
Lemon oil	Thyme oil

Put three drops of the mixture on a tissue and inhale the vapors.

For the Immune Szystem
Add fifty drops of tea tree oil to two ounces of a carrier oil and rub the mixture into your palms and the soles of your feet once a day. This will strengthen your immune system.

For Inflamed Nasal Membranes
Mix two to three drops of rose oil, chamomile oil, or lavender oil with a teaspoon of petroleum jelly and apply to your nostrils three times a day. If desired, use a combination of two or all three of the oils, but keep the *total* amount of oil you use to three drops.

For Insect Bites and Jellyfish or Sea-Urchin Stings
Add two to three drops each of tea tree oil and lavender oil to one teaspoon of alcohol or apple cider vinegar. Dip your fingertip in the mixture and dab it gently on your skin.

For Snake Bites
Apply lavender oil freely to a snake bite. Lavender oil's antiseptic and anti-inflammatory properties will treat the bite and its scent will help keep the victim calm. *Note:* Lavender oil is useful as an interim measure while awaiting medical help; it should *not* be used in place of urgent medical therapy.

ADDITIONAL WAYS TO USE ESSENTIAL OILS

There are many ways to apply essential oils to the body. In addition to the ways just described, baths, footbaths, and massage are recommended for the relief of allergy symptoms.

For a bath, add five to ten drops of one or a combination of essential oils to a tub of water. Soak in the scented water for fifteen minutes.

For a footbath, add five drops of one or a combination of essential oils to a shallow pail of hot water. Soak your feet for fifteen minutes.

For a massage, add about nineteen to twenty drops of one or a combination of essential oils to two ounces of a carrier oil. A good combination is eight drops of tea tree oil, eight drops of rosemary oil, and three drops of cinnamon leaf oil.

CONTRAINDICATIONS

Even though they are natural products, essential oils can be dangerous because they are so highly concentrated. It is important to read the labels, which, according to law, should carry precise safety data. Here are some general guidelines to follow when using essential oils:

- Avoid oils derived from plants to which you are allergic, since they can cause problems.
- Use citrus oils cautiously because they can cause sun sensitivity.
- Do not apply essential oils undiluted to the skin. Lavender

oil and tea tree oil are exceptions. Lavender oil helps the skin to heal and can be applied directly to insect bites, rashes, and even burns and cuts. Tea tree oil has effective anti-infectious, anti-inflammatory, antiseptic, antiviral, and antifungicidal properties.

- Be aware that some essential oils may interact with certain medications. While the oils are usually safe, new drugs are constantly coming on the market that may interact adversely with them.
- Keep essential oils away from the eyes.
- Avoid sweet fennel oil if you have epilepsy.
- Avoid rosemary oil, sage oil, and thyme oil if you have high blood pressure.
- Do not take undiluted essential oils by mouth because they are highly concentrated and can damage the mucous membranes of the digestive system. Some oils, pennyroyal in particular, can be highly toxic when ingested.
- Do not apply essential oils directly to a lightbulb, as they can cause the bulb to explode. There is a special ring that can be filled with an essential oil and placed on a bulb.
- Do not use clary sage oil for several hours before or after drinking any form of alcohol. It can cause nausea and exaggerate the effects of the alcohol.

Although the most common contraindications are listed, if you have any doubts about using a particular essential oil, you would be wise to consult a qualified aromatherapist.

.   .   .

Aromatherapy, like herbal therapy, represents a return to nature focusing on the well-being of the individual as a whole. Rather than being considered an alternative treatment, it should be viewed as a complementary therapy useful for relieving and reducing allergy symptoms.

6

Homeopathy

According to aerodynamic theory, bumblebees cannot fly. According to the laws of physics and chemistry, homeopathy cannot work. However, bumblebees fly and homeopathy has brought relief to countless numbers of people all over the world. Celebrities such as Lindsay Wagner, Tina Turner, and Vidal Sassoon have even publicly endorsed homeopathy.

The British royal family is among those who rely on homeopathy. Prince Charles uses *Arnica* to heal his bruises when he falls off a polo pony, and Queen Elizabeth II always travels with twenty-four homeopathic preparations. Everyone wonders what the Queen carries in that ever-present pocketbook slung over her arm. Perhaps it's those twenty-four remedies!

THE LAW OF SIMILARS

Homeopathy is based on two tenets—the Law of Similars and the Law of Infinitesimals. According to the Law of Similars, if a substance produces certain debilitating symptoms in a healthy person, then a small dose of that substance could be used to treat the same symptoms in an ill person. Immunizations and allergy shots are also based on this principle. Simply stated, like cures like.

Immunizations and allergy shots are two types of mainstream medications that are routinely given in microdose amounts. With an immunization, a tiny amount of a deactivated microorganism is given to stimulate the body's immune response. This helps protect the body from the disease that would result from exposure to a large amount of the active microorganism. Allergy shots supply minute amounts of the allergy-triggering substance to encourage the development of tolerance to larger amounts of the allergen.

The principle that homeopathy follows is similar. Rather than attempting to suppress the symptoms of a condition, it works with the symptoms to cure the condition. The fundamental principle of homeopathy is that symptoms are the body's efforts to heal disease. By using extremely diluted amounts of a substance that in a more concentrated form would make the body ill, it encourages the body's own defenses to come to the rescue.

This approach is completely opposite to that of mainstream medicine, which treats most conditions with substances designed to suppress symptoms. The idea in homeopathy is to stimulate the body's own disease-fighting mechanisms by using extremely small doses of a substance that will trigger the mechanisms and then to allow those mechanisms to do the healing.

Although the Law of Similars seems to be something like the concept behind immunizations, mainstream scientists say that the resemblance is superficial. Causing even more of a problem in the minds of mainstream doctors is the Law of Infinitesimals, which really defies scientific logic.

THE LAW OF INFINITESIMALS

The Law of Infinitesimals states that the more a remedy is diluted, the stronger its effect will be.

What is difficult for most lay people and researchers to understand about homeopathy is that, the smaller the dose, the stronger the remedy. The tenet of extreme dilution is a tremendous challenge to the laws of physics and chemistry.

Opponents of homeopathy argue that there is not enough of the substance left to do any good. Devotees, however, insist that science lacks the tools to properly assess homeopathy. Since most scientists cannot understand how an infinitesimally diluted substance can have any biologic effect, they dismiss homeopathy and argue that any results are due to the placebo effect. The placebo effect is the response to a substance caused by the patient's belief in the substance—that is, if the patient believes the substance will bring relief from symptoms, the patient feels relief. The placebo effect can also be negative, with no response noted by a patient who believes a substance is worthless.

PREPARATION OF REMEDIES

A homeopathic remedy is prepared by diluting the active ingredient in water or alcohol, shaking it, then diluting the dilution, and shaking it again. The remedy is diluted and shaken repeatedly, until hardly any of the original substance remains. The shaking process is called *succussion*. Each successive dilution and succussion is called *potentization*.

A hypothesis of homeopathy is that the shaking process releases the effects of the original substance, creating an electrochemical pattern that remains in the diluted solution and that, when the remedy is ingested, is spread throughout the system via the water in the body.

Dr. Samuel Hahnemann, a German physician and the founder of homeopathy, theorized that diluting a remedy actually makes it stronger. Dr. Hahnemann proposed the theory that vigorous shaking transfers the spiritlike essence of the medicine to the solvent and that each successive shaking makes the solution even more potent. This diluted but potent solution then stimulates healing while minimizing adverse reactions.

HISTORY OF HOMEOPATHY

Homeopathy was born out of Dr. Hahnemann's frustration with mainstream medicine as it was practiced in the latter part of the eighteenth century. Dr. Hahnemann was horrified by such therapies as bloodletting, purging, and blistering, and he left his medical practice to seek safer ways to treat his patients.

One of his investigations focused on malaria treatment. Dr. Hahnemann dosed himself with quinine (a drug still in use to this day) and noticed that he experienced the same chills and fevers symptomatic of malaria, the very disease it was supposed to cure. Besides himself, he used his seven children as guinea pigs to test his remedies. From this experiment, he formulated his Law of Similars.

Since Dr. Hahnemann was the kind of doctor who believed in minimal intervention, he wanted to determine how little of a medication could be given while still promoting healing. He began diluting his remedies by mixing one part of the active ingredient with nine parts of water or alcohol, shaking the solution vigorously, then repeating the process as many as thirty times.

Dr. Hahnemann believed that the symptoms of an illness are the result of the body's efforts to restore itself to health and that triggering those symptoms using a homeopathic remedy can stimulate the body's own defenses to cure the illness. He created the word "homeopathy" from the Greek words *homoios,* which means "like," and *pathos,* which means "suffering."

The Rise and Fall of Homeopathy

Homeopathy became quite popular in the United States during the nineteenth century. By the early part of the twentieth century, four out of every ten doctors in the United States were homeopathic physicians, and there were more than a hundred homeopathic hospitals. Then, with the advances in orthodox medicine and the introduction of drugs such as penicillin and other antibiotics, the interest in homeopathy faded, and the homeopathic healing method was pushed aside, especially in the United States.

Another reason for the decline of homeopathy was, and is, the growing power of the American Medical Association (AMA). Homeopathic facilities were forced to close when they could not receive accreditation from the AMA. However, despite the AMA's insistence on rigorous drug testing, when the current regulations were drawn up, most homeopathic remedies were already in use, so they were "grandfathered" in. Interestingly, the FDA does regulate the manufacture of homeopathic drugs.

The Revival of Homeopathy

Homeopathy, much more widely used around the world than our system of orthodox medicine, is now coming back into favor in this country for the following reasons:

- Homeopathic remedies have no side effects.
- Homeopathic remedies are easy to use.
- Homeopathic remedies work for a variety of ailments.
- Homeopathic remedies cost only a fraction of traditional remedies.

In the mid-1980s, mainstream medical journals began publishing studies supporting homeopathy. In 1986, orthodox researchers at the University of Glasgow in Scotland tested a homeopathic hay-fever remedy in a double-blind, placebo-controlled study involving 144 people with pollen allergies. The group taking the homeopathic preparation showed a significant reduction in symptoms, and their need for antihistamines was reduced by 50 percent.

During the three-year period from 1988 to 1991, the sales of homeopathic remedies grew from $11 million to $150 million. By 1995, Americans were spending more than $165 million a year for homeopathic preparations, and sales were rising by 20 to 25 percent a year. By 1996, sales reached $227 million and were increasing by 12 percent a year. At the same time, the number of homeopathic practitioners in the United States increased from 200 in 1970 to 3,000 in 1996. In the United States, about 200 physicians are also homeopathic specialists, although homeopathic practitioners do not have to be medical doctors to practice homeopathy.

THE REMEDIES

The homeopathic pharmacopoeia contains more than 2,000 remedies taken from vegetable, animal, and mineral sources. These sources include substances such as snake venom, crushed bees, and plant parts. The sources are used in minute quantities to stimulate the body's own defense and immune functions. *Oscillococcinum,* the popular flu remedy, for example, is homeopathic. A natural product that works with the body, it contains very small doses of the active ingredient *anas barbariae hepatis cordis extractum HPUS 200 CK.* The body uses only the amount of medicine it absolutely needs. The medicine has no side effects, is strong enough for adults, and is safe enough for children.

Homeopathic remedies activate the immune system without causing any kind of negative reaction. Practitioners choose a remedy based on its ability to mimic the condition. In the United States, the homeopathic remedies are prepared in FDA-approved homeopathic pharmacies, and in most parts of the world, including the United States, they are available without a prescription. In France, where homeopathy is widely accepted and practiced, pharmacies are required by law to stock homeopathic remedies.

Homeopathic remedies are available from homeopathic practitioners, over the counter at pharmacies, at health food stores, and by mail order. They are better used for chronic or minor conditions than for emergencies. The average cost of a homeopathic remedy is $6.

Homeopathic preparations are helpful for treating allergies because, in many situations, a diluted dose of the allergen can be prepared as a homeopathic remedy. For instance, diluted solutions of ragweed pollen have been shown to reduce or prevent a reaction when the supplement is given for several weeks before the start of the allergy season. This is the same principle upon which immunotherapy is based.

Even though you can obtain homeopathic preparations without a prescription, homeopathic physicians like to screen patients for dietary, environmental, mental, and emotional factors in order to prescribe the most appropriate remedy. Most homeopaths are physicians or other licensed medical professionals, and know when conventional medical care or referral to a specialist is necessary.

VISITING A HOMEOPATH

One reason people choose to consult a homeopathic physician is the more personalized care. Your first visit to a homeopath can take from one to one-and-a-half hours, and you will be surprised at how much more attention than normal you get from the practitioner. Besides your physical symptoms, the homeopath will take into consideration your emotional and mental states. He or she will take note of the way you talk and dress, and will ask you detailed questions about your moods and food cravings.

If you complain about a cough, he or she will ask you questions such as:

- Is it worse when you eat or drink?
- Do you have to hold your chest when you cough?
- Do environmental changes affect you?

Homeopaths believe in treating the whole person rather than just the illness. Whereas an orthodox physician will give two people with the same symptoms the same medicine, a homeopath will most likely give each person a different medication, taking into consideration each person's unique personality and temperament. By the time you are given a medication, you will have the feeling it was designed especially for you, rather than for your condition. Some homeopaths give only one remedy at a time, while others prescribe combinations.

READING THE LABEL

To determine how much of the original substance is in the medicine, look at the number and letter (X, C, or M; these are the Roman numerals for 10, 100, and 1,000, respectively) on the label. The lower numbers and the letter X indicate lower dosages. Remedies with a C or M are considered higher dosages, better taken while under the care of a homeopathic practitioner. Remedies in the X scale have been diluted 10 times. Remedies in the C scale have been diluted 100 times. Remedies in the M scale have been diluted 1,000 times.

When a number precedes the letter, just put that number before the zeros. For instance, "3X" means 3 times 10, which equals 30, and "3C" means 3 times 100, which equals 300. As previously explained, the law of infinitesimals states that the more a remedy is diluted, the stronger its effect will be.

The label also contains information about what the remedy contains, the types of conditions it helps, and how it should be used.

HOMEOPATHIC REMEDIES FOR ALLERGY TREATMENT

Homeopathic allergy remedies are safe and non-toxic, and are available in health food stores and some pharmacies. They are available as liquids, dried granules, and pills. They are inexpensive and can be purchased without a prescription, but a homeopathic practitioner can suggest a more individualized program.

Since homeopathic remedies and combinations of remedies are so highly individualized, for both the condition and the person, it is difficult to list them all, but following are several that are good for allergies.

For hay-fever relief, try these remedies:

- *Arsenicum album* reduces hay-fever symptoms, treats allergic symptoms such as a runny nose, and eases some types of asthma.
- *Euphrasia* helps relieve runny nose, watery eyes, and some coughs.
- *Kali bichromicum* reduces head congestion.
- *Pulsatilla* helps reduce hay-fever symptoms during an attack and is useful for easing the symptoms of asthma.
- *Sabadilla* treats symptoms such as runny nose, sneezing, and itchy eyes.
- *Wyethia* helps relieve runny nose, dry throat, and itchiness behind the nose and in the palate.

For skin-allergy relief, try these remedies:

- *Apis mellifica* helps reduce swelling following insect stings and also is useful for food-allergy reactions and itchy hives. For anaphylaxis, *Apis mellifica* has proven to be life-saving. If

you are allergic to insect stings, you might consider carrying high-potency *Apis*
- *Rhus toxicodendron* treats contact dermatitis and itching.

For asthma relief, try these remedies:

- *Pulsatilla* eases the symptoms of asthma.
- *Arsenicum album, Carbo vegetabilis, Ipecacuanha,* and *Nux vomica* can be used to relieve an asthma attack while awaiting professional help.

For complete descriptions of these and other homeopathic remedies, see a guide such as *The Complete Book of Homeopathy* by Michael Weiner (Garden City Park, New York: Avery Publishing Group, 1989, 1996).

ANSWERS TO THE CRITICS

Many mainstream medical practitioners fear that homeopathy keeps patients from seeking established treatment for serious illnesses. The critics of homeopathy maintain that any successes in homeopathic treatment are due to the placebo effect. However, homeopathic remedies have been successfully used with infants, unconscious people, and animals, who do not respond to placebos. Of all the alternative therapeutic methods, homeopathy is the one that can best be tested by randomized, controlled studies, but it is also the one that most profoundly challenges orthodox medical thinking.

A report on homeopathy in the September 20, 1997, issue of *Lancet,* a prestigious British medical journal, stated that homeopathic remedies are 66 percent more effective than no treatment at all. This is greater than the effect that would be produced by a placebo. An international team of researchers led by Dr. Wayne Jonas, director of the Office of Alternative Medicine at the National Institutes of Health (NIH), participated in this study. The team analyzed eighty-nine studies of homeopathy conducted in a randomized, placebo-controlled manner. In such a study, patients are given either the substance or an identical-looking inert substitute. Neither the patients nor the researchers know who is being given what. This eliminates the experimenters' expectations and is one of medicine's strongest tools for evaluation. The results of the NIH study undermined the hypothesis that the clinical effects of homeopathy are completely due to the placebo effect and showed instead that, in certain circumstances, homeopathy does appear to work.

SAFETY NOTE

Since homeopathic remedies are so diluted, there is very little risk of adverse side effects. In addition, as a rule, they do not interact adversely with medications recommended by orthodox doctors. However, it is always prudent to inform your doctor about other treatments you are using. Many mainstream healthcare providers also have expertise in homeopathy.

While homeopathic medicines may reduce your need for conventional medical treatment, they are not appropriate for life-threatening symptoms, such as a severe asthma attack with impaired breathing or anaphylaxis, which requires immediate emergency attention. They may be used on the way to the doctor or hospital emergency room, or in conjunction with heroic medical intervention, but they should not be used as substitutes.

Unlike orthodox medicines, which tend to mask symptoms, homeopathic medicines work with the body to reinforce the immune system. They have a high safety factor and are gaining popularity all over the world among both physicians and patients who are looking for a safe, effective solution to healing. These people believe they have found the solution in homeopathy, and you, too, may want to give it a try.

7

Acupuncture, Acupressure, and Reflexology

Acupuncture, acupressure, and reflexology are three methods that heal the body by balancing its energy flow. You are probably aware of them for pain control, and, most likely, you've heard stories of people with sports injuries or other types of muscle or skeletal pain who achieved dramatic relief. In addition to relieving aches and pains, these methods are used to treat organic problems, upper respiratory infections, high blood pressure, psychological problems, and, strange as it may seem, allergies and asthma.

ACUPUNCTURE

Acupuncture has been practiced in China for more than 2,000 years. It is used to create a smooth flow of vital energy, or *chi*, throughout the body. This is done by stimulating the points on the meridians, or pathways, that are connected to the various organs, glands, and cells in the body.

Although acupuncture is considered an alternative therapy in the United States, it is a standard treatment in China, where it is just one of the several therapies that constitute traditional Chinese medicine.

Outside of Chinese neighborhoods, acupuncture was virtually unknown in the United States until a report by *New York Times* foreign correspondent James Reston in 1971. While on assignment in China, Reston underwent an emergency appendectomy. He reported that, following the surgery, acupuncture effectively blocked his pain.

Now, articles are appearing in the scientific literature confirming acupuncture's potential benefits. Even an NIH panel has concluded that, in addition to alleviating pain and nausea, acupuncture is probably effective at treating several other medical symptoms.

There is no downside to acupuncture other than its expense. A session usually costs between $75 and $100.

Both physicians and non-physicians practice acupuncture. In the United States, 4,000 of the 10,000 licensed acupuncturists are medical doctors. Americans visit both kinds of acupuncturists 12 million times a year.

How Acupuncture Works

Chinese traditional medicine views sickness as an imbalance in one or more of the electromagnetic fields in the body and brain. The theory is that the body is electrical in nature, with positive and negative poles, and that the two poles should be in balance. When the complementary life forces in the body, called *yin* and *yang,* are balanced, energy flows smoothly along the fourteen interconnected primary meridians on each side of the body. If the balance is disrupted, sickness can occur. Restore the balance, and the disease or symptom often disappears.

The meridians, each of which services one or more specific body areas or organs, are close to the body's surface at 360 different points. Acupuncturists can correct an imbalance between the yin and yang by stimulating the appropriate points. They do this by inserting tiny steel needles into the specific points related to the particular illness or symptom. This helps the body's energy to become evenly dispersed instead of remaining blocked. Balance is restored, and the body can heal itself.

Acupuncture is incomprehensible to doctors trained in orthodox Western medicine because it has not been subjected to the documentation they demand before accepting a treatment. Some orthodox practitioners have voiced the opinion that acupuncture works best in suggestible individuals and that these individuals would do just as well with hypnosis.

Practitioners of traditional Chinese medicine think it is nonproductive to spend time, money, and resources to convince Western doctors of something that has been used successfully for thousands of years. Those who believe in acupuncture point to the fact that veterinarians get very positive results using acupuncture on animals, who are obviously not affected by the power of suggestion.

Visiting an Acupuncturist

When you visit an acupuncturist, he or she will look at the condition of your *chi* to check if it is balanced. First, the acupuncturist will take your health history and question you about your digestion, diet, and sleeping habits. You also may be asked questions about your work, your energy level at various times of the day, and the temperatures that make you feel most comfortable.

The acupuncturist will then assess your situation by:

- Checking your pulse in three different places on your arm, using different degrees of pressure, to search for energy blockages in corresponding organs.
- Inspecting the color of your tongue.
- Examining your skin for eruptions.
- Noticing how you smell, since specific body odors often indicate certain disorders.
- Checking the tone of your voice, since it is a clue to your emotional state.

After assessing your particular situation, your acupuncturist will work to open your channels of blocked energy by inserting needles into the appropriate meridians in your body. This will not hurt. All you will feel, if anything, is a slight sting similar to an insect bite. The needles, made of stainless steel with copper or plastic handles, are very thin; some are as thin as a hair. The therapist will insert them to a depth of about a quarter of an inch, may twirl or twist them for a few minutes, and will then leave them in place for five to thirty minutes. Sometimes, the needles will be stimulated with a weak electrical current or heated with a burning herb. Heating the needle with a burning herb, a healing technique that originated in China, intensifies the effect of the acupuncture.

Some people with allergies notice results very quickly when treated with acupuncture, while other people experience a more gradual improvement. Many asthmatics treated with acupuncture find that they no longer need as much medication.

Acupuncture probably helps relieve asthma by:

- Working directly on the nerves, reducing their spasmodic tendency to contract when the least little irritant is present.
- Opening narrowed blood vessels in the lungs.
- Encouraging relaxation and fuller breathing.

Some insurance companies cover acupuncture treatments if they are recommended by a licensed medical doctor. To find a physician who practices acupuncture, call the American Academy of Medical Acupuncture at 800–521–2262.

Note: Although most acupuncturists use disposable needles, always make sure that your acupuncturist does, since reusable needles carry a risk of infection.

ACUPRESSURE

Acupressure is similar to acupuncture in that its aim is to balance the body's energy. Instead of inserting needles, acupressure practitioners use their fingertips to stimulate *acupoints.* Acupressure is a slower process than acupuncture and requires more repetition, but, like acupuncture, its beneficial effects result from the release of blocked energy. Many practitioners incorporate massage into their acupressure treatments. They manipulate the specific acupoints on the various meridians in the body and may press them for a period of time, usually about a minute.

When pressure is applied to an acupoint, the point may be tender, indicating a problem or energy leak connected with the organ it represents. By maintaining the pressure on the contact point, the practitioner stops the energy leak. When the leak is stopped, the polarity is reversed, and the energy can flow back to the body part that is affected. Generally, the energy flow is complete when there no longer is any tenderness at the contact point.

Most allergic symptoms, such as sneezing, a stuffy nose, headache, and teary, itchy eyes, are treated by applying pressure to the head, neck, and nose areas. Acupressure is not as powerful as acupuncture, but it can provide real benefits for many conditions, and it can be used for self-care.

Michael Reed Gach, PhD, director of the Acupressure Institute in Berkeley, California, suggests the following self-help approach to treating an allergy attack:

1. At the onset of an attack, apply pressure to the center of the webbing in your hand, between the thumb and index finger.
2. Angle the pressure towards the bone in your hand that connects with the index finger.
3. Maintain constant pressure for at least two minutes while taking slow, deep breaths.
4. Repeat the process with your other hand.

For the past fifteen years, Dr. Randy Coleman, a naturopathic doctor based in Philadelphia, has treated more than a thousand patients for allergies using acupressure and has had an

80-to-85-percent success rate. His method is to stimulate pressure points around the face to clear the meridians and remove pockets of congestion that have become stagnant. In conjunction with this treatment, Dr. Coleman does a form of soft-tissue massage in the areas around the sinuses and throat to aid in the lymphatic drainage.

REFLEXOLOGY

Reflexology is the science that deals with the principle that there are reflexes in the feet related to all the organs and body parts. Reflexologists believe that stimulating these reflexes can help many health problems. They therefore apply pressure to these points to break up deposits of waste material and to open up nerve impulses. Massaging specific areas on the feet eases problems in the corresponding parts of the body and restores the energy flow to the body's many different systems and functions. A tender spot on the foot indicates a point of congestion in the energy lines and a problem in the corresponding area.

You can use reflexology for self-treatment. For example, the pads of the toes are the sinus reflexes and massaging them often helps clear up a stuffy nose. The fleshy part on the balls of the feet under the third and fourth toes relates to the lungs and bronchial tubes. Applying pressure to this area can help to overcome an asthma attack.

When you visit a reflexologist, the treatment is not necessarily symptom-oriented. Most reflexologists do not concentrate immediately on the distressed zone. Instead, they first try to achieve a state of balance in the body in general.

You are probably familiar with the term *shiatsu*, which is another type of deep massage, based on unblocking and energizing the meridians. In case you are worried that one type of treatment can counteract another, since the body points stimulated in reflexology, shiatsu, and acupressure are similar but not all the same, please be reassured. As Ray Pierce, a massage therapist and certified practitioner and teacher of reflexology from Rockledge, Pennsylvania, says, "The theory behind all energy work is to balance the body's energy, and one form will not contradict another because everything works together to achieve optimum health."

If this chapter has helped you gain some understanding of how the energy in your body behaves, then the material presented in the next one will not seem quite as bizarre.

8

Nambudripad's Allergy Elimination Techniques

Suppose your orthodox doctor has told you that your beloved pet is the cause of your allergies. Or, perhaps testing has determined that you have to give up most of your favorite foods because of the allergic reactions you suffer from eating them. What if there was a treatment that could detect your allergies by testing the strength in your arm while you held a bit of the allergic substance? What if you could then eliminate the allergies for good with a fifteen-minute acupuncture or acupressure treatment? You'd probably want to give it a try—much to the chagrin of your orthodox doctor—wouldn't you?

When something sounds too good to be true, it usually is. However, practitioners who use Nambudripad's Allergy Elimination Techniques (NAET) say that the system works 80 to 90 percent of the time and that their patients are ecstatic with the results. NAET is a revolutionary treatment for all kinds of allergies. It eliminates reactions not only to foods, but to chemicals, plants, and animal dander. You don't have to give up your pet! All you have to do is hold some of your pet's fur while you have an acupuncture or acupressure treatment.

In addition to being a treatment for allergies, NAET also is used as a therapy for headaches, arthritis, backaches, digestive disorders, musculoskeletal disorders, hyperactivity, insomnia, chronic fatigue syndrome (CFS), premenstrual syndrome (PMS), and many other health problems. However, we will limit our discussion here to the use of NAET for food and environmental allergies.

DEFINITION OF NAET

Named for Dr. Devi S. Nambudripad, the holistic practitioner who developed the technique in the 1980s, NAET is a method of retraining the brain and nervous system to stop reacting to allergens. Orthodox medicine cannot cure allergies. All it can do is identify them and recommend strict avoidance of the offending substances. NAET, on the other hand, is a method of permanent allergy desensitization, says Dr. Nambudripad.

The NAET theory is that, if the brain has developed patterns of responses that are inappropriate and interprets an innocuous substance as harmful, the body "freezes up" its vital energy to defend against the perceived unsuitable substance. This "freezing up" of energy leads to a blockage in one or more of the body's meridians, which, in turn, results in a weakening of the immune system and body functions. An allergy is then created, and the body becomes unbalanced and symptoms appear.

NAET reprograms the brain to perceive unsuitable energies as suitable and to use them in a beneficial manner instead of allowing them to cause energy blockages and imbalances. After identifying an offending substance, NAET clears the body so it no longer reacts to the substance.

In addition to eliminating food allergies, environmental allergies, and chemical sensitivities, the technique also can be used to treat the malabsorption of vitamins and other nutrients.

HISTORY OF NAET

Dr. Devi Nambudripad is a chiropractor, acupuncturist, and registered nurse practicing in California who stumbled across her techniques accidentally. For several years, she had such severe reactions to so many foods that she was forced to exist solely on white rice and broccoli. As soon as she attempted to eat other foods, her symptoms would return. One day, even though she knew she was allergic to carrots, she nibbled on one and had an immediate and very severe reaction. Afterwards, when she gave herself an acupuncture treatment, she wondered why she felt so vitally energized and was surprised to find that a piece of the carrot had stuck to her skin. Since she was studying acupuncture at the time and knew how the body's energy behaved, she realized that something had happened to change the way her body responded to the energy field of the carrot.

Dr. Nambudripad did a muscle-response test on herself, found that she was no longer allergic to carrots, and surmised that she could begin eating them again without suffering a reaction. Following this breakthrough, Dr. Nambudripad spent several years working on her theory and has been using it on patients since 1986. She has taught the method to more than a thousand healthcare practitioners worldwide, and currently, NAET is practiced by physicians, nurses, chiropractors, acupuncturists, and, at times, even patients themselves.

THEORY OF NAET

The premise of NAET is that everything, including human beings, consists of energy. Allergies are caused by energy blockages in the body, which occur when the body comes in contact with an allergen and the body's energy field clashes with that of the allergen. The brain identifies the allergen as a clashing energy field and alerts the immune system, which responds with antibodies.

According to Dr. Nambudripad, this inappropriate reaction can cause more than the typical allergic response. It also can cause a tired feeling, headache, depression, digestive problems, and skin rashes, and can eventually lead to diseases in the vital organs. When NAET is performed and the blockages are released, the body is reprogrammed not to react to innocuous substances as if they were dangerous.

To understand the theory behind NAET, look upon the body as an energy system that consists of electromagnetic pathways connected to organs and cells. When you encounter something you are allergic to, the result can be blockages in these pathways.

This is a little easier to understand if you are familiar with the chiropractic theory that, when the spine or a bone is misaligned, nerve conduction in the body is interrupted, which in turn can lead to disease. When the misalignment is corrected, the proper balance is restored and the energy can once again flow unimpeded through the nervous system to the brain.

According to NAET theory, when energy flows freely along the meridians, allergic reaction is not possible. However, if the immune system responds to a harmless substance as if it were a threat—that is, treats a tourist like a terrorist—a blockage will occur. The immune system will cause an *autoimmune reaction,* resulting in healthy tissue becoming inflamed. This inflammatory reaction will block the energy flow along the meridians and prevent the vital energy from going to where it is needed by the system.

NAET uses the principals of chiropractic care, acupuncture, and kinesiology to bring about permanent desensitization to allergens. When an allergen is held within the energy field while acupressure or acupuncture is performed on specific areas along the spine, the antigen-antibody complex reaction is neutralized and the energy begins to again flow freely along the meridians. When the energy blockage is cleared, the brain is sent a message that the body has been desensitized to the particular allergen. From then on, since the body no longer identifies that substance as an allergen, it no longer creates energy blockages in response to it. The body has relearned how to respond to the substance—that is, learned to treat it as a tourist, not a terrorist.

MUSCLE-RESPONSE TESTING

NAET practitioners use a process known as *applied kinesiology,* or muscle-response testing, to determine allergies to particular substances. This test identifies blockages in the energy field by testing muscular strength.

Generally, the test is performed using the arm. While lying down, you will be asked to extend your arm at a 90-degree angle, palm facing outward. The practitioner will try to establish your strength by pushing the extended arm toward your foot while you resist. Then, while you hold the food or other substance being tested in your other hand, the practitioner will push the extended arm again to see if the muscle has become weakened. If your arm is weakened and the practitioner can push it, the chances are great that you are allergic to the substance you are holding. If your arm remains strong, you are most likely not allergic to the substance. Some practitioners use a computerized electroacupuncture device that measures even tiny changes in electrical response through the skin. This device can be used to test for hundreds of foods in one session without tiring your arm.

Muscle-response testing yields the same result for allergies and hypersensitivities, and allergic individuals are treated the same way as those who are hypersensitive. This is because NAET theory holds that both allergies and intolerances can compromise the immune system, lower resistance, and cause a predisposition to colds and other ailments.

Muscle-response testing is widely discredited by orthodox doctors, who find it difficult to believe that pushing against an arm can reveal a food allergy. Its proponents say that it works because the physical body responds to extremely subtle changes in the energy field. Even though scientific evidence is lacking, growing anecdotal evidence is pointing to the efficacy of NAET therapy in treating allergies.

Surrogate Testing

Muscle-response testing also can be performed by surrogate on infants, children, animals, the very sick, and the physically incapacitated or debilitated. If possible, the person being tested should hold the suspected allergen. If this is not possible, the allergen can be loosely strapped to the test subject's skin or, in the case of animals, worn in the collar.

While the surrogate touches the individual being tested, the practitioner tests the muscle response of the surrogate. As the subject's energy flows through the surrogate, any weakening is reflected in the surrogate's body.

Self-Testing

Muscle-response testing also can be done on a self-test basis Although testing done by a trained professional is more accurate, self-testing can often help in an emergency and is quick and easy to accomplish. Here's how it's done:

1. With one hand, touch your little finger to your thumb to make a circle.
2. Using the index finger of your other hand, try to separate the little finger and thumb. Unless you have carpal tunnel syndrome or a structural problem, you should not be able to separate the fingers.
3. To test a substance, hold a small amount of it in the palm of the hand with which you are making the circle and try again to separate the fingers. If you are allergic to the substance, your fingers will be weakened and come apart.

The self-test form of muscle-response testing is especially useful if you know you have food allergies and want to quickly test for a particular food before eating it.

TREATMENT WITH NAET

To achieve permanent relief from your allergies, your central nervous system has to be reprogrammed to sense allergens in a new way. If you are allergic to a tested substance, a strong muscle will weaken in response to a message from your brain. Your practitioner will then use acupuncture or acupressure while you hold the allergen, or a vial containing a solution of the allergen, in your energy field. This will free the blocked energy and reprogram your nervous system to learn a different response.

After the treatment, you will have to avoid the offending substance for twenty-five hours. This means:

- You must not eat the food.
- You must not come within four feet of the food.
- You must not inhale the food if it is being cooked.

Failure to follow this twenty-five-hour avoidance rule may cause you to lose the benefit of the treatment, and you will have to repeat the process. However, if you do adhere to the rule, you, like most people, will find that your body has been retrained to accept the formerly offending substance without creating an energy blockage. In other words, your allergy will be completely and permanently gone.

NAET also can be used to treat occupational allergies to substances such as paint, gas and diesel fumes, chemicals in the workplace, hair dyes, and photographic chemicals. Even sick-building syndrome can be treated. After Craig R. started a new job in a sealed building, his skin started to itch and tingle. He had previously been tested for food allergies, so he knew which foods to avoid and cut them out of his diet. He also switched laundry detergents. However, he still found no relief. Luckily, he mentioned his problem to his chiropractor, who happened to be a NAET practitioner. The chiropractor had Craig collect some of the air in his office in a bottle and gave him a NAET treatment using it. The treatment worked, and Craig's problem is now permanently gone.

THE NAET PROTOCOL

Most people don't understand why NAET practitioners follow the same initial protocol with all patients rather than just treating each patient for what ails him or her specifically. All NAET practitioners start with the same series of ten basic treatments for the most common allergies.

The ten basic treatments address the essential nutrients the body needs for its normal physiological and emotional functions. These nutrients usually are absorbed from food, but someone who is allergic to a food can't absorb the nutrients from that food. For instance, if you are allergic to eggs, you cannot absorb the nutrients, such as protein, from eggs.

Clearing

The process called *clearing* is not the same as desensitizing. Rather, clearing is a method of reeducating the nervous system. Dr. Nambudripad says it is important to "clear the elements" in the order she recommends. First, the body is cleared 100 percent of the top ten elements. In 80 to 90 percent of patients, other allergies go away after just the first five elements are cleared. This is because the clearing process reduces the stress on the immune system and allows the body to function better.

Patients can be tested and treated for thirty groups of basic food and environmental items in an order prescribed by Dr. Nambudripad. Dr. Nambudripad bases her prescribed order on the items' importance to the body. Clearing these basic allergens in the proper sequence is necessary for success. The theory is that clearing the basic ten groups first strengthens the immune system. The basic nutrients are those nutrients that are essential for the body's functioning. Once the body can utilize the basic nutrients properly, health will improve. The list includes the foods that are the most allergenic, and the vitamins and minerals found in them.

Usually, one treatment per week is recommended. Some people take two treatments a week. Even though you may be among the few to overcome an allergy in just minutes or, in some cases, hours, the majority of cases, as previously stated, take twenty-five hours to clear. If you aren't among the people able to clear rapidly and are exposed to an allergen sooner than allowed, the treatment will be nullified and you will need to go through it again. This is not something most people want to do because, in addition to the extra time involved, the treatments cost from $40 to $60 per visit.

The Mixes

The NAET Guide Book, written by Dr. Nambudripad as the companion workbook to her original *Say Goodbye to Illness,* lists seventy-two foods and twenty-four environmental items. The first five food mixes, also called "elements," are as follows:

1. Egg mix—includes eggs, chicken, feathers, and the antibiotic tetracycline, since it is commonly given to chickens. This element is cleared first because these products are

common ingredients in many foods, vitamins, and cosmetics.

2. Calcium mix—includes all dairy products, most root and green vegetables, sesame and sunflower seeds, oats, navy and dried beans, soybeans, almonds, walnuts, peanuts, sardines and salmon, and, of course, calcium supplements.

3. Vitamin-C mix—includes fresh fruits and vegetables, juices, soft drinks, milk, artificial sweeteners, and vitamin-C supplements.

4. Vitamin-B mix—includes whole grains, fruits, vegetables, meat, dairy products, and anything containing the B vitamins. *Note:* People with severe allergies may have to be tested and treated for each B vitamin individually.

5. Sugar mix—includes all food and nonfood products containing sugar from any source (for example, cane sugar, honey, molasses).

The next five elements are the iron mix; vitamin-A mix, including fish and shellfish; mineral mix; salt mix; and corn mix.

After treating for the basics, most practitioners muscle test for each element once again to make sure that all of them have been cleared.

BENEFITS OF CLEARING

Very often, when a patient is treated for one allergy, another allergy is cleared. For instance, many patients report that, after being cleared for the first five mixes, they are no longer sensitive to ragweed. Being treated for a mold allergy sometimes clears allergies to dried fruits and nuts. Treatment for a gluten allergy can clear allergies to the grains that contain gluten—wheat, rye, oats, malt, and barley.

Clearing for sulfites, the material used to preserve wine and prevent salads from discoloring, often clears allergies to foods such as avocados, dried fruits, shrimp, cider, commercially baked goods, gelatin, potatoes, vegetables, salad, wine, and beer. Ironically, sulfites are frequently used in the manufacture of drugs and asthma aerosols.

Eczema and acne also respond to NAET. Eczema in children is usually caused by an allergy to wheat, corn, or the B vitamins. In adults, eczema can be caused by an allergy to food, clothing, animals, chemicals, fungi, yeast, or bacteria.

When children have eczema, they are highly likely to be allergic to the B vitamins and to foods containing them, and this may be a precursor of a wheat allergy. Eliminating any allergies to the B vitamins or to wheat will usually clear up the eczema and may prevent the later onset of asthma.

Treating for a corn allergy can clear up a myriad of other allergies, since corn is hidden in so many products besides food. In her book, *Winning the War Against Asthma and Allergies,* Dr. Ellen Cutler lists some 200 food and nonfood products containing corn.

FOOD CRAVINGS

The reason people crave the foods to which they are allergic is that the allergy prevents them from properly absorbing the food, thereby causing a deficiency in the nutrients the food contains.

Alcoholics might be allergic to an ingredient in alcoholic beverages, such as sugar, grapes, brewer's yeast, malt, corn, or the B vitamins. The same holds true for overweight people because an allergy to their favorite foods might cause intense cravings for the foods.

NUMBER OF TREATMENTS

The amount of time it takes to treat a chronic condition with NAET varies from person to person. You cannot eliminate all of your allergies in one or two office visits. Some patients have to be treated as often as three times a week for one or two years, depending on their immune-system response. Patients with milder allergies may complete their treatments in two or three months. The average amount of time it takes is eight to twelve months.

In her book, *Say Goodbye to Illness,* Dr. Nambudripad says statistics show that 80 to 90 percent of the allergic patients who receive proper NAET treatments are either entirely relieved or satisfactorily improved. It is not a quick fix, but those who are willing to take the time and who have the financial resources usually experience vast permanent improvement.

SELF-TREATMENT WITH NAET

Self-treatment with NAET is possible while awaiting medical treatment. Stimulating specific acupressure points while holding the allergen may help reduce or even eliminate symptoms. Although self-treatment with NAET is not a substitute for an emergency allergy kit, which contains antihistamines and injectable epinephrine, it is a useful adjunct. Ask your practitioner to show you where the acupressure points appropriate to your condition are located.

TWENTY-FIVE-HOUR RULE

Patients often question why it is necessary to keep away from the allergy-causing substance for twenty-five hours. The reason is that it takes twenty-four hours for energy to circulate through all the meridians—two hours for each of the twelve meridians. So, to be on the safe side and to make sure the blockages have cleared, NAET practitioners add one hour, bringing the waiting period to a total of twenty-five hours.

Patients are instructed to shop before the treatment for the foods they are allowed to eat during the twenty-five-hour period. This is because if they shop after the treatment, they could inhale or come in contact with a substance that could cause a reaction and render the treatment invalid.

During the twenty-five-hour treatment period, both the patient's diet and environment must be strictly controlled. For instance, during treatment for the first mix, eggs, chicken, and tetracycline must be avoided. Not only must all foods containing these products be avoided, but also all shampoos and cosmetics containing egg products, as well as anything made with feathers, such as pillows and down quilts.

Clearing for the B-complex involves more than testing for and clearing the supplements. All foods containing the various B vitamins, such as whole grains, fruits, vegetables, meat, and dairy products, must be avoided. So many foods contain the B vitamins, in fact, that some people find it necessary to live on Jell-O and tapioca pudding prepared with water for the twenty-five hours. People severely allergic to the B vitamins sometimes need to be treated for each B vitamin separately.

People being cleared for the mineral mix are instructed not to eat or touch root vegetables, use or touch metals of any kind, or drink or bathe in tap water. They must avoid wearing jewelry and need to wear gloves if they have to come in contact with a metal surface. They are required to use glassware for cooking and plastic utensils for eating.

Many practitioners also suggest avoiding hot showers, overactivity, and anything that excites the body negatively or positively in order not to overstimulate the autonomic nervous system during the twenty-five-hour period. Although the restrictions may seem very prohibitive at first, they are not all that difficult to follow, since only one restricted regimen is followed, and for just twenty-five hours, following each treatment.

While patients who cheat and don't follow the twenty-five-hour rule have to repeat the treatment, those who are not exposed to the allergen during that time period should expect to be desensitized.

CASE HISTORIES

Cassandra, a yoga teacher, noticed that she was not getting tanned in the sun and was getting a lot of insect bites. After eating, she would break out in hives, first on her elbows and then all over her body. She scratched so much that she developed strep and staph infections with a lot of pus. Desperate, she contacted a NAET therapist. In addition to clearing her for the first ten mixes, the practitioner put a scraping of her skin in a test tube and cleared her for that. It took six months of treatments once or twice a week, but in the end, her skin was completely cleared. Her husband was so impressed with her positive results that he also took the treatments, which cleared his environmental allergies and sugar cravings.

Paula, a dance teacher with a master's degree in microbiology and infection control, injured her knee while skiing. When she refused surgery, the orthopedic surgeon who recommended it said, "You'll be back to me." Paula instead went for acupuncture and noticed an improvement in two weeks. She is now 95 percent better, but, of course, the disbelieving orthopedic surgeon insisted the knee healed itself.

While being treated for the knee injury, Paula mentioned that she bruised easily, even though her platelet count was normal, and that she always became sick at Christmastime because of the Christmas trees. The acupuncturist, who was also a NAET practitioner, performed tests that showed she was not utilizing vitamins B, C, and E properly and also was reacting to chicken. Paula was cleared for all these substances and has not had a problem since.

After having had her allergies cleared by NAET, Kitty sought help for her children. She had been advised that her three-year-old son should have a tonsillectomy, but the experience had been so bad for her older son that she decided to try NAET instead. Once her younger son was cleared for the calcium mix, he showed remarkable improvement and stopped waking up five or six times a night. As a result, it was determined that he no longer needed a tonsillectomy. As a beneficial side effect of the treatment, the boy's feet, which had been turned in, were straightened. Kitty was even more thrilled by the NAET results on her older son. The older boy had had episodes of violence and had been diagnosed with Tourette's syndrome. Even strict adherence to the Feingold diet (which eliminates the consumption of all foods with additives, coloring agents, or chemicals) didn't help. But once the boy was cleared for the corn mix, his violent tendencies subsided. Now, he can drink soda, is no longer allergic to dogs, and is like a "regular kid," according to his mother.

ANIMALS

A good number of veterinarians use NAET. Like all alternative practitioners, these veterinarians say that orthodox medicine only suppresses symptoms, has side effects, and doesn't cure allergies. Their alternative approach is to get to the cause of the problem and correct it, and their treatments provide permanent elimination of allergies in 80 to 90 percent of the animals they treat. To test and treat an animal, the vet puts the mixes into vials and ties the vials around the animal's neck.

Many allergies are obvious because they cause itching, coughing, and sneezing. Others cause small, barely noticeable dysfunctions that can later evolve into major health problems. Allergy sensitivities can lead to skin problems, ear problems, gastrointestinal problems, eye problems, and respiratory problems, among others. Some practitioners of both humans and animals subscribe to the theory that more than a hundred conditions are caused by allergy sensitivities. They believe that eliminating the underlying allergies will improve the patient's overall health and well-being—whether the patient is human or animal.

Animals, like humans, are tested and treated for the ten basic mixes, as well as for substances from their diet and environment. Following identification of the offending allergen, the animal is treated with acupressure, which retrains the animal's body to treat the offending substance as a friend, not a foe. Like a human, the animal must avoid the allergen for twenty-five hours following treatment. The animal's owner is given a list of items that have to be avoided during this period. For instance, a dog with a grass allergy will have to be kept off the lawn and, depending on its size, carried or driven to a grassless area to exercise and eliminate.

. . .

The theory of how NAET works is difficult for most lay people—and nearly impossible for orthodox doctors—to accept. Orthodox doctors say that no controlled studies have ever been done to document that NAET works. Yet, the success rate of the therapy is between 80 and 90 percent of all patients treated. Many holistic practitioners became aware of NAET while pursuing treatment for their own or their child's severe allergies. In addition to chiropractors and licensed acupuncturists, some osteopathic physicians and even some medical doctors now treat with NAET.

You can find a listing of NAET practitioners in Dr. Ellen Cutler's book *Winning the War Against Asthma and Allergies.* She includes about 200, by state or province, in the United States and Canada. If you have Internet access, the website <www.naet.com> has a directory of practitioners by geographic area.

Visual Imagery

Close your eyes and, in your mind, picture an orange. Pick up the orange, lightly scratch its skin, and sniff it. Then, take a knife, put the orange on a cutting board, and cut it in half. Pick up one of the halves and squeeze a few drops of juice onto your tongue. In all likelihood, you are now salivating. This is guided visual imagery, and you have just practiced it.

Now, think of something that scares you, perhaps something like a bridge or an elevator, and imagine yourself crossing that bridge or being stuck in the elevator. More than likely, your heart is beating faster than normal now and your blood pressure has risen. Again, you have just practiced guided visual imagery.

We may not be aware of it, but guided imagery is something we all do. If you have ever worried about something (and who hasn't?), you've used guided imagery. It's a method of seeing, hearing, smelling, and tasting things in your imagination that evokes a physical response. The images might come from interaction with a therapist (interactive guided imagery), from a cassette tape, or even from something you read.

Various forms of guided imagery are currently in popular use, and they all are beginning to gain scientific credence. The following are some of the conditions for which they are useful:

- Controlling pain
- Shrinking tumors
- Healing persistent infections
- Overcoming sleep disorders
- Reducing hyperactivity
- Expanding creativity
- Self-healing of all types

Guided imagery used before surgery has helped patients recover faster and with less pain. Cancer patients using the technique have found that it stimulated their immune systems.

ALLERGIES AND THE MIND

The peptide receptors in the cells of the immune system are the same as those in the cells of the brain, a fact that enables us to communicate with ourselves. If thinking of an orange can make you salivate and imagining something that scares you can increase your heart rate and blood pressure, then picturing yourself healthy can free you of allergy symptoms.

It is possible to actually have an allergy attack just by reenacting within yourself a time you had one. People with hay fever, for example, can see a field of goldenrod blowing in the wind on a television screen and find their noses starting to run and their heads becoming stuffed up.

The importance of the mind in relation to asthma and allergies has been thoroughly documented. There was one case in which a patient with a severe allergy to roses had a major attack just from having a fake rose placed near him. Dr. William Mundy, clinical professor of medicine at the University of Missouri School of Medicine, Kansas City, has a friend with an allergy to flowers. This friend went to a museum and, while looking at glass flowers in a glass case, had a terrible allergic reaction. Merely alerting his immune system that he was in the presence of flowers, even glass ones, caused the reaction.

HISTORY OF VISUAL IMAGERY

Guided imagery was developed in the 1970s to help athletes and musicians perform better. Studies have shown that basketball players who visualize their shots do just as well as those who actually practice them. In recent years, research has established that the mind can communicate instructions to the cells in the body that influence the onset and outcome of illness. These studies have shown that relaxation techniques and imagery can affect the body's physiology and enhance the immune system. Clinical experience has shown that almost everyone can benefit from imagery.

Many cancer patients become interested in imagery as a technique to help rid themselves of the disease. In their minds, they picture the cancer cells as something being destroyed by something else. For instance, they may visualize their immune system as soldiers with ray guns and the cancer cells as the enemies being zapped.

Experts agree that visual communication with the immune system works best. Although it is possible to talk to the immune system or have feelings about it, it seems to pick up best on visual images. The important thing is to find images that help you visualize. For allergy relief, try imagining yourself surrounded by a pollen-free atmosphere or the inside of your nose being cleansed by clear, pure protective fluid. See your membranes change from deep red to pale pink and picture your swollen tissues shrinking. As you picture it, so it can happen.

CAUSES OF ALLERGIES

To comprehend how visualization works to stop the allergy process, it helps to understand what causes allergies. The theory behind mind-body allergy treatment is that the cells of the immune system respond to allergens according to instructions received from the brain. In other words, the nervous system and immune system communicate with each other. Therefore, if the brain signals the immune cells to produce IgE and attack a harmless substance mistaken for a harmful substance, that substance is treated as harmful and attacked whenever it enters the body from that time forward. Based on this theory, it is believed that people can learn to reprogram the messages that their brains send to their immune cells.

Ordinarily, when a harmless substance, such as pollen or animal dander, gets into the system, it is gobbled up by special cells called macrophages and filtered out through the lymph system. But, if the harmless substance comes into the system at the same time as a virus or bacteria, the body may form antibodies to it. The immune system might not be able to tell the difference between the harmless substance and the virus or bacteria, and in its zeal to do a good job, it tries to fight off *all* the extraneous particles. So, from that time forward, whenever the harmless substance enters the body again, the immune cells mistakenly read it as a harmful substance and attack it, causing the immune system to respond. The mucous membranes become swollen and inflamed, and the skin probably erupts as well.

The immune system is set up so that when something menacing such as bacteria or a virus comes in, it puts a little marker (like a red flag) on the dangerous cells. You may once have had a sore throat or mild viral infection (not necessarily anything serious) and, while sick, inhaled something harmless you had been inhaling for years, such as ragweed or some kind of pollen. In trying to do a good job and not wanting to make a mistake, your immune system rushed out and also tackled the harmless substance. An immune battle ensued, with a lot of histamine being released at the battle site. This was the immune system doing its best to keep anything from harming you, even substances with no intrinsic harm.

THE VISUALIZATION PROCESS

There are a number of visualization techniques, but the most specific for allergy control are those developed by William L. Mundy, MD. Dr. Mundy has been teaching medical students and residents at the University of Missouri School of Medicine since 1949. In addition, he has maintained a private practice specializing in psychosomatic disease, internal medicine, and psychotherapy. Originally a conventionally trained physician, Dr. Mundy's interest and expertise in psychosomatic disease and in the work of healers in areas outside of conventional medicine have paved the way for him to deal with allergy patients in a unique way.

Dr. Mundy believes that visual imagery, as opposed to auditory suggestion or other similar techniques, works the best with the immune system. Most of the time, Dr. Mundy teaches his patients a process known as *reframing,* which is based on the theory that if you can change how you perceive an event, you can alter its course.

Visualization is much less expensive than other methods and does not have side effects. You can do it with your eyes open or closed and at any time you wish. Even though it can be used effectively by most people, it is not a good idea to practice it while engaged in something such as driving. In addition, people with severe asthma suffering from allergies should consult with their physicians before discontinuing their allergy medication.

According to Dr. Mundy, visual imagery done with the help of a therapist has an 80-to-90-percent success rate. He likens the technique to chicken soup, saying, "If it doesn't help, it won't hurt." Just like anything new that is learned, it must be practiced and done a little at a time. It would be foolhardy for someone with a dust allergy to try the technique once and then walk through a whirling dust storm. The more the visualization process is practiced, the better the immune system will relearn, or reframe, its responses.

CASE HISTORIES

To illustrate how visual imagery works, following are several case histories representing a cross-section of allergies that can be helped by the technique. The method used was similar in all the cases, whether the patient was being treated for a mold, airborne, pollen, or animal-dander allergy, or a lactose intolerance. Note that in all cases, a safety factor, usually an imaginary Plexiglas shield, was used to protect patients from having an attack while visualizing themselves in the allergic situation.

Mold and Fungus Allergy

Joan suffered from an allergy to mold for six years. Whenever she was exposed to mold, she developed a low-grade fever and fatigue, sometimes accompanied by a cough. She traveled frequently with her husband and often reacted to the mold in hotel and motel bathrooms. Here is how Dr. Mundy treated her:

> *Dr. Mundy*: "Imagine you are someplace where you get that allergy, and experience it for a moment. Try to picture in your mind what a fungus looks like."
>
> *Joan*: "Mold in bathrooms. The black stuff around the faucets that hasn't been scrubbed off."
>
> *Dr. Mundy*: "Think of something similar to mold that doesn't set off your allergy, something that you find pleasant."

Joan: "Maybe caviar. I like caviar, and that does not give me a reaction."

Dr. Mundy: "We are going to put up a thick Plexiglas wall between you over here and an image of yourself on the other side of that wall. Look at yourself on the other side of the wall thinking of having a fancy caviar hors d'oeuvre. See yourself looking at and inhaling the odor of caviar while you are breathing comfortably. Notice how pleasant the fragrance of the caviar is."

Joan breathes comfortably and easily.

Dr. Mundy: "Now, bring in just a few particles of the moldy stuff you saw in the hotel bathroom, and watch the Joan on the other side of the Plexiglas shield as the moldy particles gradually mix with the caviar and she continues to breathe comfortably and easily, without any allergic symptoms. See how her system allows her to take a healthy inhalation and know that this combination is perfectly safe and she has no reason to react in an unhealthy fashion.

"Gradually increase the amount of mold you mix with the caviar, and notice how your entire respiratory tract is comfortable and how the mixture is perfectly easy for your body to manage. Check your inner self to make sure you are comfortable watching this scene. Next, put a plastic bubble around the Joan on the other side of the screen and a plastic bubble on the Joan over here. Lift the Plexiglas screen and slowly bring the bubble with the Joan over there to where you are sitting over here in your bubble. Just as soap bubbles enter each other's space and join each other, bring that bubble from over there and let it meld with the bubble around the you over here.

"Notice how comfortable it is to breathe around those things that used to be a problem for you. And let your immune system know you thank it for being aware that there is no reason to be concerned and that you can manage those things in a comfortable, healthy physiologic way."

Dr. Mundy then instructed Joan to respect her immune system and to be careful not to overload it. For instance, he cautioned that it would not be wise for her to go into a basement full of moldy books, which often irritates even people without a mold allergy. In addition, he instructed her to repeat the process in her mind a few times each day in a quiet place.

Airborne Allergy

Judy reacted to the type of airborne particles that blow around in dry areas on windy days. Since this reaction occurred mostly in summertime, it was referred to as hay fever. Her nose would run, and she would cough up huge amounts of phlegm. Here is how Dr. Mundy treated her:

> *Dr. Mundy:* "Think of a place you can go where you don't have that seasonal airborne allergy, a place where you can be without having an allergic response to airborne particles."
>
> *Judy:* "I can breathe without difficulty when I am near pine trees."
>
> *Dr. Mundy:* "Let's put up a Plexiglas shield, and see Judy over there taking nice deep easy breaths in a pine forest and see how comfortable she is. Watch her over there as some of the air, laden with the particles that caused a

problem in the past, comes near her. Do these particles have a color or a particular shape to them?"

Judy: "I see them as skinny inch-long pieces of dust flying in the air, and they are sort of a yellowish-beige color."

Dr. Mundy: "Bring a small handful of some of those yellowish particles into the pine forest and let them mix with the air over there. Notice how comfortably you are breathing this mixture. Now, gradually increase the amount of these skinny yellow particles you are mixing with the pine-scented air as you continue to breathe easily. Do you feel good over there?"

Judy: "My nose itches."

Dr. Mundy: "It may be that anyone subjected to too much stuff might need to use a handkerchief. They might have to cover their face if exposed to too much dust. You have to respect your immune system and give it a little help. Now, put a bubble around the Judy over there and imagine her in the bubble breathing comfortably in the pine forest. Put a bubble around the Judy over here, lift the Plexiglas wall, and let the bubble from over there meld with the one over here. Go through this process several times a day, letting your immune system know that the other particles are harmless tourists and that you can continue to feel good."

Dr. Mundy told Judy to repeat the process and gradually increase her exposure to the airborne particles. He cautioned her not to overload her immune system prematurely because, even though patients sometimes experience dramatic relief, it is not a good idea to rush the process.

Pollen Allergy

Sam had a seasonal allergy for twelve years. It usually started in the middle of August and lasted until the first frost. Standard tests showed that it was an allergy to ragweed and pollen. Here is how Dr. Mundy treated Sam:

Dr. Mundy: "Imagine you were having an allergic response to the pollen. See yourself and become aware of how you felt. Your eyes may begin to water. You can even think of an advertisement for a cold medicine on television that has someone with a runny nose. Put yourself in that scene, and your nose may start to run.

"Now, try to remember a place you have been where you were breathing comfortably and enjoying the air, perhaps the seashore or the mountains."

Sam: "I like the ocean. I feel good there and can breathe well."

Dr. Mundy: "Put a thick Plexiglas shield in front of you that completely blocks you off. Look through it and visualize yourself on the seashore. Your eyes can be open or shut. Remember how good the sea smells and how comfortably you are breathing and what an overall good feeling you have. Now imagine there are particles in the air that you and anyone else can smell. Let's call them sea particles. What color would they be?"

Sam: "Kind of brown, smelling good."

Dr. Mundy: "Imagine inhaling these wonderful sea particles and how much you enjoy having them circulate through your lungs, your capillary walls, your entire body, and notice how great everything feels. Experience that for a few minutes and then tell me what the ragweed and pollen particles look like."

Sam: "Tiny stuff with prickles on them, sort of grayish-brown prickly things."

Dr. Mundy: "Now imagine another scene about twenty feet away from the wonderful, comfortable beach scene and put into that scene a little cloud of the gray-brown ragweed and pollen things. Very slowly bring the cloud closer and introduce just about a tablespoon of that cloud at a time into the wonderful sea air you are breathing so comfortably. Watch the tablespoon of the pollen cloud dilute and disappear into the sea air. All you now sense, know, smell, feel, and are sure of is that you are breathing in particles that are comfortable for you to manage.

"Now reach out and take more, perhaps a little handful, of that cloud, bring it over, and watch how the sea air dilutes it and dissolves it so you can't see the difference anymore. Keep on bringing in as much as you want of the cloud of prickly gray-browns, a little at a time, and recognize now that your body knows it can handle those things, that they are simply tourists, that they are of no danger, and that they can circulate through your system very comfortably.

"Because we need to respect and honor our immune system, ask it if it feels comfortable in this new process. Maybe it will answer you and tell you it doesn't have to overact anymore. It doesn't have to exert any energies in that direction, and it thanks you for telling it. Look inside your lungs and blood vessels, and realize everything is fine in there and you are breathing in a way that is pleasant, easy, and comfortable for you.

"Think of blowing soap bubbles, and put a bubble around the you on the shore who is breathing so well and comfortably, and who has no more problems with the gray-brown prickles. Put a bubble around the you over here. Now, lift up the Plexiglas shield and bring that bubble from the other side towards you and watch one bubble melding into another. Here comes the bubble with you breathing so well and so comfortably, and it touches you sitting here, becomes one with you, surrounds you, and becomes a part of you. Is that comfortable for you to visualize?"

Sam says yes, and Dr. Mundy instructs him to repeat the process several times a day.

Animal Dander

Ann had two cats and wanted to keep them, but she was allergic to cat dander and developed severe eye symptoms. Here is how Dr. Mundy treated her:

Dr. Mundy: "What can you picture in your mind that is similar to cat dander but does not affect you?"

Ann: "Dust doesn't bother me at all."

Dr. Mundy: "Imagine dust on a stuffed animal that is very much like the dander. Put up the Plexiglas shield and visualize yourself on the other side with the dusty stuffed animal. See yourself with it, feeling good and breathing comfortably. About twenty feet away, visualize a cloud of dander, and bring over about a tablespoon of it at a time and mix it with the dust on the stuffed animal and the dust in the house, and see it passing comfortably through your system. Picture yourself feeling well and happy with the stuffed animal and the cat dander. Whenever you feel ready, imagine the cat coming over and sitting with you and the stuffed animal.

"Put a bubble around yourself over here and another one around the you with the stuffed animal on the other side of the Plexiglas shield. Lift the screen and bring the bubble over here, and let it slowly surround you, meld with you, and become one with you. Notice how comfortable and happy you are, and realize that your properly functioning immune system will continue to make you happy. Ask your immune system how it feels, and talk to it as you review this process in your mind for the next several days."

It would not have been prudent for Ann to play with a cat or have one sit on her lap right after the treatment. Instead, she increased her exposure gradually by spending more and more time in a house where there was a cat.

Although some patients experience dramatic relief, all are cautioned to respect their immune system and not overload it too soon.

Lactose Intolerance

The process used to treat lactose intolerance is different from what is normally used to treat allergies. For lactose intolerance, a system known as *anchoring* is used. An *anchor* is a stimulus that is paired with a highly predictable set of responses. The pairing usually does not make any sense to the rational mind, although the phenomenon is universal in human behavior. The process of anchoring is intended to cause a deliberate association between a stimulus and a particular experience. Anchors can be kinesthetic, auditory, visual, or foreground/background, and they do not require constant reinforcement to be effective. Below is an example of *foreground/background anchoring.*

Sara had suffered from lactose intolerance since childhood. Here is how Dr. Mundy treated her:

Dr. Mundy: "Think of what you can swallow and enjoy that is similar to lactose."

Sara: "I can drink soy milk. It looks like regular milk."

Dr. Mundy: "Imagine yourself drinking soy milk and enjoying it. What do your feet feel like in your shoes now?"

Sara: "They are tingling."

Dr. Mundy: "Imagine how you felt in the past when you were drinking regular milk."

Sara: "It's like a sharp knife twisting in my stomach. Even a small amount of milk in my cereal can make me feel bloated."

Dr. Mundy: "We have chosen a scene in the foreground that is something pleasant, like drinking soy milk. Now we bring in something from the background which you have been aware of, like the tingling feeling of your feet in your shoes. When we do this, it often happens that the foreground you brought back will overwhelm the reaction you had prior to the experiment. There are times when people can't remember anymore how the allergic reaction felt."

While Sara was in a positive state (imagining herself drinking soy milk), her attention was directed to another state (the tingling in her feet). These two states therefore became paired in her mind. When the negative state (drinking cow's milk) was brought into the foreground, her nervous system anchored that to the positive background (the tingling feet), too. This happened because the nervous system cannot be in two incompatible states at the same time—for example, you cannot feel hot and cold at the same time. As a result, the old pattern was broken and a new one created.

The other kind of anchoring commonly used is called *kinesthetic anchoring*. This type of anchoring involves touch. The following is an example of kinesthetic anchoring:

Dr. Mundy (sitting in front of Sara with a hand on her knee): "Imagine yourself having that bad lactose response. Nod your head when you remember how bad you feel and maybe even bring up some of the symptoms."

Sara: Nods.

Dr. Mundy (putting his other hand on her arm): "Now imagine yourself with the soy milk that you are drinking with comfort and pleasure. Nod your head when you feel it."

Sara: Nods.

Dr. Mundy (lifting both hands): "Now try to imagine the lactose-milk scene."

Sara says that she is having a problem recalling the scene because it is no longer in her memory.

What Dr. Mundy did was apply a kinesthetic anchor by putting one hand on Sara's knee while having her visualize a bad reaction. Then he put his other hand on her arm and had her visualize a good reaction. Finally, he collapsed both anchors by taking both hands away at the same time, thus anchoring her mind to the positive reaction. Anchors also can be visual or auditory, but kinesthetic anchors seem to be the most powerful.

Sara reported that after one night, she was able to eat many things she had not been able to touch since childhood, such as blue cheese. She could even use milk on her cereal. Anchoring is hard to do alone, however, and usually requires the assistance of a therapist.

SELF-HELP

Think of yourself as a cartoonist and imagine what the allergic particles that have been a problem to you in the past might look like under a microscope. How would they appear if you could draw them in three dimensions and color? Keep that picture in your mind and place an imaginary six-inch-thick Plexiglas wall in front of you, one you can see through but that still keeps you completely separated from what is on the other side. Since you are completely separated, you won't have to react to what you see over there.

See another you on the other side of the Plexiglas wall and imagine that the person you see over there is having an allergy attack. Around the other you are the little particles you drew, and the other you is experiencing the symptoms of your allergy while in the presence of those particles. Next, leave the you having the allergy attack and think of a place where your breathing is not a problem and where you feel good, maybe the seashore or the mountains. See particles there that you can inhale and swallow. They smell and taste good, and you feel healthy. See the particles mix pleasantly with your breathing and then circulate through your bloodstream.

Now, see the other you, the one having the allergic reaction, and see the cloud of allergic particles around that you. Reach out and take a small handful of the allergic particles and bring them back to the you that is surrounded by the healthy particles and feeling so good. Notice how the allergic particles simply disappear in the midst of the pleasant ones. Keep reaching over and bringing back more and more handfuls and watch them disappear. Then, take a bucket and bring back a lot of the particles and see how they no longer are a problem. Watch them mix with all the pleasant particles that you are able to inhale and enjoy. You have blended the allergic you with the healthy you and the resulting you no longer has a reason to be concerned with the particles that used to be a problem.

See the now-healthy you on the other side of the Plexiglas wall encased in a pleasant, colorful bubble. Next, imagine the you on this side of the wall also encased in a bubble. Lift up the wall and watch the bubble from over there come to the bubble over here. Watch as the bubble from over there meets the one over here and how the two bubbles become one, just as two soap bubbles meet and blend into one. See your body no longer having any problem with the particles that have now been made harmless and are simply a part of what your body handles all the time. See and feel every part of your body become free of the things that used to bother you. Go through this process several times a day in your mind and you will retrain your immune system.

Dr. Mundy has a number of testimonials from professionals who have used his technique on themselves to overcome their allergies. Some had to listen to the two tapes that accompany his book three to four times a week, and others had to listen just once. One woman with severe allergies to dog and cat dander used the tapes for only one day and was able to play with her neighbor's dog and cat the next day without experiencing any allergic symptoms at all.

Some patients have been cured of multiple allergies within hours. One physician healed herself of allergies to dust, mold, animal dander, yeast, wheat, dairy, and citrus products within one day. Another woman cured herself of a lifelong lactose intolerance in a few hours.

Visual imagery has been successfully used in treating almost all kinds of allergies. Many people can simply listen to the process being utilized with someone else and can then use it to cure themselves.

You don't have to understand or even believe in the mind-body connection. All you have to do is be interested enough to try the approach and experience the results that are almost universally excellent in telling the immune cells to stop hyperreacting.

Conclusion

You have the right, as a member of a free society, to be an active participant in deciding which healthcare path you wish to pursue. Being aware of your options should help you in this decision and should make you a better-informed consumer when it comes to your well-being. To this end, I have tried to give you impartial information about several different alternative allergy treatments, some tried and true, others relatively new on the scene.

Granted, it is difficult to determine which treatment or combination of treatments is best for you. The ideal situation would be to find a nutritionally oriented medical doctor who is also a homeopath with NAET training and adept at visualization techniques. Such a "full-spectrum" practitioner could evaluate which methods would be best for treating *you*. However, in this age of super-specialization, where everyone knows more and more about less and less, it is unlikely that any one person could be well versed in all these treatment methods. Perhaps someday, in the not-too-distant future, a facility will exist where all these types of practitioners will cooperate with each other and work together. It could be structured like the orthopedic centers that have on staff a surgeon, a physical therapist, a chiropractor, and a massage therapist. Until that day comes, however, it behooves you to be as well informed as possible about all the allergy treatments that are available and to take an active part in your treatment.

It is not the purpose of this book to denigrate orthodox medicine or to overly praise any alternative therapy. It is no doubt true that many orthodox practitioners resist changing the way they treat allergies because it is difficult to change a lifetime of training. And, of course, there are times—such as when anaphylaxis, shock, or another emergency situation threatens your life—that it would be foolhardy not to use conventional medicine. Orthodox medicine does excel in emergency situations. When you call the founder of NAET and reach her answering machine, even her message says, "If this is an emergency, go to an emergency room."

The American Medical Association is beginning to recognize that more and more Americans are turning to alternative medical treatment, even though they almost always have to pay for it themselves. In November 1998, at least eighty articles on alternative therapies were published in scientific journals, something that was unthinkable ten years ago. I hope this book has provided you with enough information to educate yourself and to help you select the best treatment for your allergies. Good luck—and here's to your allergy-free future.

Advantages and Disadvantages of Treatment Methods

All allergy treatments have positive and negative aspects. Following is a listing of the advantages and disadvantages, as well as the cost factor, of each treatment discussed in this book.

ACUPUNCTURE, ACUPRESSURE, AND REFLEXOLOGY

Advantages: They have a balancing effect on the entire body. They can be used in conjunction with other treatments.

Disadvantages: They have no appreciable disadvantages.

Cost factor: Moderate to high. They are usually not covered by insurance.

AROMATHERAPY

Advantages: It is easy and pleasant to use. Essential oils have a regulating effect, calming or stimulating the body according to its needs.

Disadvantages: Most essential oils can irritate the skin if applied undiluted. Some can interact with certain medications.

Cost factor: Moderate. It is rarely covered by insurance.

CONVENTIONAL TREATMENTS

Allergy Shots

Advantages: They can be effective at preventing and controlling symptoms.

Disadvantages: A course of treatment is time-consuming, expensive, and uncomfortable. The side effects include the potential for anaphylaxis.

Cost factor: High. They may be covered by insurance.

Antihistamines

Advantages: They reduce and relieve symptoms.

Disadvantages: They are not a cure. They have side effects ranging from simple, such as dryness, to serious, such as the potential for fatal interactions with other drugs.

Cost factor: Moderate. They may be covered by insurance.

Avoidance

Advantages: It works very well. It is considered the ideal solution.

Disadvantages: It is time-consuming and difficult to do.

Cost factor: Minimal.

Bronchodilators

Advantages: They relieve acute allergy attacks.

Disadvantages: Their side effects include the potential for increasing the heart rate, elevating the blood pressure, and causing insomnia and anxiety.

Cost factor: Moderate. They may be covered by insurance.

Cortisone

Advantages: It can give dramatic relief from allergy symptoms.

Disadvantages: It is relatively safe in the short term, but in the long term, it can cause the immune system to become suppressed.

Cost factor: Moderate. It may be covered by insurance.

Cromolyn

Advantages: It is an effective preventive measure if started in advance of the allergy season.

Disadvantages: It is ineffective for acute attacks. It takes time to work.

Cost factor: Moderate. It may be covered by insurance.

Decongestants

Advantages: They relieve stuffiness. They ease breathing.

Disadvantages: They have side effects, including the potential for raising the blood pressure.

Cost factor: Moderate. They may be covered by insurance.

HERBAL THERAPY

Advantages: It addresses the underlying problem. It eliminates the cause of a problem rather than suppressing the symptoms. With the exception of ephedra, which should be used only under supervision, herbs have few side effects.

Disadvantages: It takes time to work.

Cost factor: Minimal.

HOMEOPATHY

Advantages: It works with symptoms rather than fighting them. It stimulates the immune system and encourages the body to heal itself. It has no side effects. It is easy to use. It can be used for self-treatment.

Disadvantages: It has no appreciable disadvantages.

Cost factor: Minimal. Visits to practitioners may be covered by insurance.

NAMBUDRIPAD'S ALLERGY ELIMINATION TECHNIQUE (NAET)

Advantages: It has a high rate of efficacy. About 80 to 90 percent of patients find relief from their allergy symptoms. It has no negative side effects. It often causes improvement in non-allergy conditions as well. It is useful for a wide variety of problems.

Disadvantages: It is time-consuming and expensive.

Cost factor: High. It is usually not covered by insurance.

NUTRITIONAL THERAPY

Advantages: It is safe and effective. It strengthens the entire system. It has no side effects, but supervision is recommended when taking megadoses of any individual nutrient to avoid creating deficiencies in others.

Disadvantages: It is not a quick fix. It takes time to work. Some diets are restrictive and difficult to follow.

Cost factor: Minimal to moderate.

VISUAL IMAGERY

Advantages: It has no side effects. It can be done either with a therapist or alone. It has a 90-percent success rate when done with a therapist.

Disadvantages: It has no appreciable disadvantages.

Cost factor: Minimal for self-treatment. Moderate to high for treatment with a therapist. It may be covered by insurance.

APPENDIX B

Resource Organizations

The following organizations can provide you with information on specific allergies, disorders, and/or therapies. Note that the addresses and telephone numbers are subject to change.

Allergy and Asthma Network, Mothers of Asthmatics
3554 Chain Bridge Road
Suite 200
Fairfax, Virginia 22030
800–878–4403

American Academy of Allergy, Asthma and Immunology
600 East Wells Street
Milwaukee, Wisconsin 53202
800–822–ASMA
http://www.aaaai.org

American Association of Oriental Medicine
433 Front Street
Catasaqua, Pennsylvania 18032
610–266–1433

American College of Allergy, Asthma and Immunology
85 West Algonquin Road
Suite 550
Arlington Heights, Illinois 60005
800–842–7777

Asthma and Allergy Foundation of America
1125 15th Street, NW
Suite 502
Washington, DC 20036
800–7–ASTHMA

Food Allergy Network
10400 Eaton Place
Suite 107
Fairfax, Virginia 22030
703–691–3179
http://www.foodallergy.org

Herb Research Foundation
1007 Pearl Street
Suite 200
Boulder, Colorado 80302
303–449–2265

Homeopathic Educational Series
2124B Kittridge Street
Berkeley, California 94704
510–649–1294

IAQ (Indoor Air Quality) INFO
PO Box 37133
Washington, DC 20013
800–438–4318
http://www.epa.gov/IAQ

Lung Line
800–222–LUNG

National Center for Homeopathy
801 North Fairfax Street
Suite 306
Alexandria, Virginia 22314
703–548–7790
http://www.homeopathic.com

National Jewish Medical and Research Center
1400 Jackson Street
Denver, Colorado 80206
800–423–8891
http://www.njc.org

Office of Alternative Medicine Clearinghouse
PO Box 8218
Silver Spring, Maryland 20007
888–644–6226
http://altmed.od.nih.gov

Parents of Asthmatic/Allergic Children
1412 Marathon Drive
Fort Collins, Colorado 80524
303–842–7395

Bibliography

BOOKS

Balch, James, and Phyllis Balch. *Prescription for Nutritional Healing, Second Edition.* Garden City Park, NY: Avery Publishing Group, 1997.

Burton Goldberg Group. *Alternative Medicine: The Definitive Guide.* Puyallup, WA: Future Medicine Publishing, 1993.

Castleman, Michael. *Nature's Cures.* Emmaus, PA: Rodale Press, 1996.

Credit, Larry P., Sharon G. Hurtunian, and Margaret J. Nowak. *Your Guide to Complementary Medicine.* Garden City Park, NY: Avery Publishing Group, 1998.

Cutler, Ellen. *Winning the War Against Asthma and Allergies.* Albany, NY: Delmar, 1998.

Fezler, William. *Imagery for Healing, Knowledge and Power.* New York: Simon and Schuster, 1990.

Houston, Francis M. *The Healing Benefits of Acupressure.* New Canaan, CT: Keats Publishing, 1991.

Kastner, Mark. *Alternative Healing.* La Mesa, CA: Halcyon Publishing, 1993.

Lankton, Steve. *Practical Magic.* Capitola, CA: Meta Publications, 1980.

Lawless, Julia. *The Complete Illustrated Guide to Aromatherapy.* New York: Barnes and Noble, 1997.

Lee, William H. *Aromatherapy for the Nineties.* New Canaan, CT: Keats Publishing, 1991.

Lupkowitz, Myron A., and Tova Navarra. *Allergies A-Z.* New York: Facts on File, 1994.

Moore, Thomas J. *Prescription for Disaster.* New York: Simon and Schuster, 1998.

Mundy, William L. *Curing Allergies With Visual Imagery.* Shawnee Mission, KA: Mundy and Associates, 1993.

Murray, Michael. *Natural Alternatives to Over-the-Counter and Prescription Drugs.* New York: William Morrow and Co., 1994.

Nambudripad, Devi S. *The NAET Guide Book.* Buena Park, CA: Delta Publishing, 1996.

Nambudripad, Devi S. *Say Goodbye to Illness.* Buena Park, CA: Delta Publishing, 1993.

Novick, Nelson Lee. *You Can Do Something About Your Allergies.* New York: Macmillan Publishing Co., 1994.

Page, Linda. *How to Be Your Own Herbal Pharmacist.* Sonora, CA: Healthy Healing Publishers, 1997.

Panos, Heimlich. *Homeopathic Medicine at Home.* Los Angeles, CA: J.P. Tarcher, 1980.

Pressman, Alan, Herbert D. Goodman, and Rachelle Nones. *Treating Asthma, Allergies and Food Sensitivities.* New York: Berkley Publishing Group, 1997.

Rosenfeld, Isadore. *Dr. Rosenfeld's Guide to Alternative Medicine.* New York: Random House, 1996.

Rossman, Martin. *Healing Yourself.* New York: Walker and Co., 1987.

Samuels, Michael. *Healing With the Mind's Eye.* New York: Summit Books, 1990.

Sheldrake, Rupert. *Seven Experiments That Could Change the World.* New York: Riverhead Books, 1995.

Simonton, O. Carl, Stephanie Matthews-Simonton, and James L. Creighton. *Getting Well Again.* New York: Bantam, 1992.

Wagner, Edward M., and Sylvia Goldfarb. *How to Stay Out of the Doctor's Office: An Encyclopedia for Alternative Healing.* New York: Instant Improvement, 1992.

Wagner, Edward M., and Sylvia Goldfarb. *Your Body's Most Powerful Healers.* New York: Instant Improvement, 1996.

ARTICLES

Avalon, Bruce B. "Homeopathy for Homesteaders." *Mother Earth News,* 14 April 1998, pg. 16.

Chillot, Rick. "Homeopathy: Help or Hype." *Prevention,* Vol. 50, pp. 106–109.

Cimons, Marlene. "Seldane Pulled for a Safer Allergy Drug." *Los Angeles Times,* 30 December 1997, pg. A-1.

Cole, Wendy, and D. Blake Hallanan. "Is Homeopathy Good Medicine?" *Time,* 25 September 1995, pg. 47.

Fern, Jessica. "Which Natural Medicine Is for You?" *Natural Health,* March/April 1998, pp. 119–124.

Gaby, Alan R. "New Ways of Becoming Allergic." *Townsend Letter for Doctors and Patients.* August/September 1996, pg. 128.

Hellmich, Nanci. "Docs Seek Handle on Herbs." *USA Today,* 25 November 1997, pg. 01-A.

Howe, Maggy. "Country Remedies." *Country Living,* Vol. 17, pp. 60–62.

Kai, Mauree. "Farewell to Allergies With NAET." *Progressive Health,* Fall/Winter 1997, pp. 1, 10.

Kaye, Lauren. "Natural Remedies: An Alternative to Drugs." *Metro West Jewish News,* 27 July 1995.

McKenna, M.A.J. "Sense Soothing Aromatherapy Gains Ground." *Atlanta Journal and Constitution,* 15 May 1997, pg. F-03.

Mandelbaum-Schmid, Judith. "Alternative Approaches." *Self,* April 1998, pg. 101.

Marston, Wendy. "Gut Reactions." *Newsweek,* 17 November 1997, pg. 95.

Mead, Nathaniel. "Mind/Body Answer to Allergies." *Natural Health,* October 1995, pp. 58–64.

Nightingale, Charles. "Treating Allergic Rhinitis With Second Generation Antihistamines." *Pharmacotherapy,* Vol. 6, No. 5, pp. 905–914.

Noble-London, Kate. "Health: Tried the Live Sardine Cure?" *Time,* 1 September 1997, pg. 37.

Rosen, James P. "ABC's of Allergy Testing." *Food Allergy News,* August 1997, pg. 1.

Sampson, Hugh. "Food Allergy." *Journal of the American Medical Association,* 10 December 1997, pg. 1893.

Segal, Marian. "Anaphylaxis: An Allergic Reaction That Can Kill." *FDA Consumer,* 1 May 1998, pp. 21–23.

Stovsky, Renee. "A Healthy Difference." *St. Louis Post Dispatch,* 18 April 1993, pg. 01-C.

Wallis, Claudia. "Why New Age Medicine Is Catching On." *Time,* 4 November 1991, pg. 68.

Weber, Linda. "The Man Who Couldn't Lift a Pea." *Natural Health,* July/August 1998, pp. 107–182.

Weil, Andrew. "Relicving Hay Fever." *Self Healing,* Vol. 1, No. 1, pg. 6.

INDEX

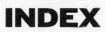

allergies (*cont.*)
   life-threatening, 6, 11, 13, 16, 18, 28, 36,
      94–95
   symptoms of, 5, 7, 9, 10–11, 15, 17, 102
allergists, 23
American Academy of Medical
      Acupuncture, 101
American Medical Association (AMA),
      87–88, 144
anaphylactic shock, 6, 17, 36, 37–38, 92,
      94–95
anchoring, 136–139
angelica, 62
animals, 99
   dander of, 9, 10, 24–25, 36, 105, 106, 116,
      135–136
   NAET and, 110, 111, 121
antibiotics, 13–14, 16, 31–32, 72, 114
antibodies, 72, 108, 127
   immunoglobulins, 6, 8, 12, 36, 62, 64,
      69
antigens, 6, 7
antihistamines, 21, 29–32, 33, 45, 52, 148
antioxidants, 44, 45, 47–51, 54, 65
   synthetic, 28
Apis mellifica, 92–93
applied kinesiology, *see* muscle-response
      testing
arachidonic acid, 41–42, 64
Arnica, 83
aromatherapy, 71–82, 148
   absorption in, 73, 75, 77–78, 79, 80
   for asthma, 77
   in baths, 73, 80
   for congestion, 76–77
   contraindications in, 80–81
   for hay fever, 78–79
   history of, 72–73
   for immune system, 79
   for inflamed nasal membranes, 79
   inhalation in, 72, 73, 74–75, 76–77,
      78–79
   for skin allergies, 77–78
   for snake bites, 79
   for stings, 79

Arsenicum album, 92, 93
astemizole, 31, 32
asthma, 8, 11, 17, 34–35, 37, 41, 42, 44, 48,
      52, 53, 58, 62, 63, 66, 94, 103, 116,
      125, 128
   acupuncture for, 97, 101
   aromatherapy for, 77
   homeopathic remedies for, 93
   see also bronchodilators
autoimmune reactions, 109
avocados, 27, 47, 55, 116
avoidance, 15, 24–29, 38, 106, 149
   of contactants, 26
   of ingestants, 27–28
   of inhalants, 24–25
   of injectants, 28–29
ayurvedic herbalism, 69

barley water, 40
basil oil, 78
baths, 67, 73, 80
bay leaves, 27
bayberry, 62
Beals, Mark G., xiii–xiv, xv
bee pollen, 46–47
Benadryl, 30, 37
benzoin oil, 77
beta-carotene, 46, 54–55
bioflavonoids, 40, 41, 45, 61
black currant oil, 67
black pepper, 69
black walnut, 67
blood testing, 21–22
blue gum oil, 76, 78
brain, 8, 108, 109, 124–127
   NAET and, 106–107
   scents and, 72, 74
Braly, James, 16, 62
brazil nuts, 27, 50
Brethine, 35
Bricanyl, 35
bromelain, 46
brompheniramine, 30
bronchodilators, 35, 149
   natural, 40, 41, 62, 63

Bronkometer, 35
burdock, 48, 54, 67

cajeput oil, 78
calcium, 46, 115
calendula, 67
cancer, 46, 48, 54, 124, 126
Candida albicans, 34
candidiasis, 16, 34
capsaicin, 40, 62
Carbo vegetabilis, 93
carotenoids, 54
carrier oils, 75, 79
cats, 9, 10, 135–136
cayenne pepper, 40, 48, 54, 62, 69
cellular allergy, 6
ceterizine, 31
chalk, 9
chamomile oil, 77, 78, 79
Charles, Prince of Wales, 83
chemicals, 10, 12–13, 44, 106, 112, 116
chi (vital energy), 98, 99, 100
chicken, 16, 50, 118
chickweed, 48, 54, 67
China, 60
    acupuncture in, 98, 99, 101
chiropractic, 108–109, 113
Claritin, 31
chlorpheniramine, 30
Chlor-Trimeton, 30
citrus rinds, 40
clary sage oil, 77, 78, 81
cleaning products, 9, 10, 12, 26, 112–113
clinical immunologists, 23
clove oil, 72, 78
coffee, 40, 43
cold extract, preparation of, 67
Coleman, Randy, 102–103
Complete Book of Homeopathy, The (Weiner), 93
congestion, 9, 15, 40, 62
    aromatherapy for, 76–77
    see also decongestants
contact dermatitis, 15, 21, 67
contactants, 10–11
    avoidance of, 26

Coricidin, 30
corn, 16, 17, 27, 55, 115, 116
cortisone, 33–34, 52, 149
cosmetics, 9, 10, 26, 115, 118
Coumadin, 49
cravings, food, 116–117
cromolyn, 34–35, 45, 46, 149
Cutler, Ellen, 116, 122
cypress oil, 77

dairy products, 16, 41, 43, 50, 55, 115, 118
dander, animal, 9, 10, 24–25, 36, 105, 106,
        116, 135–136
death, 6, 13, 38
decoction, preparation of, 67
decongestants, 33, 63, 149
    dietary, 40–41
    essential oils, 74, 76–77
    herbal, 65, 66
De materia medica (Dioscorides), 60
depression, 17, 55, 108
detergents, 10, 26, 112–113
dietary modification, 39, 40–44
    adding foods and beverages in, 40–42
    avoiding foods and beverages in, 41–42
    Murray diet in, 42–44
Dimetapp, 30
Dioscorides, Pedanius, 60
diphenhydramine, 30
Drixoral, 30
dust, 9
dust mites, 20, 24–25, 36

eczema, 15–16, 17, 21, 67
    aromatherapy for, 77–78
    NAET and, 116
eggs, 16, 43, 51, 52, 114–115, 118
Egypt, ancient, 34, 60
elder, 62
elimination diet, 19
Elizabeth II, Queen of England, 83–84
emergency measures, 37–38, 41, 117
environmental factors, 12–13, 44
ephedra, 62–64
ephedrine, 62–63

ma huang, 62–63
magnesium, 46, 55–56, 64
malaria, 86–87
marjoram oil, 77, 78
massage, 73, 75, 80, 101–102
    reflexology, 97, 103–104
mast cells, 8, 28, 41, 44, 45, 64
Maxair, 35
medications, 57, 60, 73
    allergenic, 11, 13–14, 16
medications, therapeutic, 21–22, 29–36,
        38, 41, 42, 58, 59, 61, 66, 128
    antihistamines, 21, 29–32, 33, 45, 52
    bronchodilators, 35
    cortisone, 33–34
    cromolyn, 34–35, 45, 46
    decongestants, 33
    interactions of, 31–32, 81
Medihaler-Iso, 35
melissa oil, 77, 78
melons, 27, 42
metals, 9, 118–119
mind, 124–127
molds, 9, 11, 20, 24–25, 36, 41, 42, 115,
        129–131
mucus-forming foods, 41, 42
mullein, 54, 65
Mundy, William L., xv, 7, 14–15, 125, 128,
        129–139, 140–141
Murray, Michael, 42–44
muscle-response testing (applied kinesi-
        ology), 107, 109–111, 112, 121
    self-testing in, 111
    surrogate testing in, 110–111
myrrh, 65
myrrh oil, 78
myrtle oil, 78

NAET Guide Book, The (Nambudripad), 114
Nambudripad, Devi S., 106, 107–108, 113,
        117
Nambudripad's Allergy Elimination
        Techniques (NAET), 105–122, 150
    animals and, 110, 111, 121

case histories of, 112–113, 119–120
clearing in, 113–114, 115–116
cost of, 114
definition of, 106–107
effectiveness of, 122
history of, 107–108
mixes in, 114–115, 118–119, 121
muscle-response testing in, 107,
        109–111, 112, 121
number of treatments with, 117
protocol of, 113–115
self-treatment with, 117
theory of, 108–109
treatment with, 112–119, 121
twenty-five-hour rule in, 112, 114,
        118–119, 121
Nasalchrom, 34
National Institutes of Health (NIH), 94,
        98
Neosinephrine, 33
nutmeg oil, 72
nutrition, 10, 13, 14, 16, 18, 19
nutritional supplementation, 39,
        44–57
    bee pollen, 46–47
    beta-carotene, 46, 54–55
    buying of, 56–57
    magnesium, 55–56, 64
    quercetin, 41, 45–46
    RDAs of, 56
    safety of, 57
    selenium, 44, 50–51
    vitamin-B complex, 46, 51–54, 64
    vitamin C, 44, 45, 46, 47–49, 53, 64
    vitamin E, 44, 49–51, 53
nutritional therapy, 14, 39–58, 151
    see also dietary modification; nutri-
        tional supplementation
nuts, 16, 27, 49, 50, 55, 115
Nux vomica, 93

onions, 41, 45, 48, 50, 69
Oregon grape, 67
Ornade, 33